D1216328

# MORAL ISSUES IN HEALTH CARE

An Introduction
to Medical Ethics

# MORAL ISSUES IN HEALTH CARE

## An Introduction to Medical Ethics

**Terrance C. McConnell**
University of North Carolina at Greensboro

**Wadsworth Health Sciences Division**
Monterey, California

**Library of Congress Cataloging in Publication Data**

McConnell, Terrance C.
   Moral issues in health care.

   Includes bibliographies and index.
   1. Medical ethics.   I. Title.
R724.M292       174'.2       81-16283
ISBN 0-534-01134-9          AACR2

Copyright © 1982 by Wadsworth, Inc.,
Belmont, California 94002.
All rights reserved. No part of this book may be
reproduced, stored in a retrieval system, or tran-
scribed, in any form or by any means—electronic,
mechanical, photocopying, recording, or otherwise—without the prior written permission of the
publisher, Wadsworth Health Sciences Division,
Monterey, California 93940, a division of
Wadsworth, Inc.

Printed in the United States of America

10   9   8   7   6   5   4   3   2   1

Subject Editor: James Keating
Production Coordinator: Stacey Sawyer
Manuscript Editor: Allan Graubard
Production Editor: Project Publishing & Design, Inc.
Cover design: Albert Burkhardt
Interior design: Jay's Publishers Services, Inc. and
                  Project Publishing & Design, Inc.
Typesetting: Project Publishing & Design, Inc.

# Preface

This textbook in medical ethics grew out of my experience in teaching such a course at the University of North Carolina at Greensboro. I found that, although there are many excellent anthologies used in medical ethics courses, there are no books that summarize the major positions on the principal issues in the field. Consequently, there is a serious problem in assigning readings for students. Most of the articles in anthologies were originally written for professional journals and are difficult for many undergraduates to master. What students need, I believe, is a general framework in which they can place these advanced and sometimes technical writings. This book provides such a framework. It can be used as the main text in a course on biomedical ethics, or it can provide a supplement to any of the major anthologies; it may also be used in conjunction with case studies material.

Because of widespread disagreement that exists in the field, one might think that there is no such thing as textbook knowledge in medical ethics. However, in philosophical matters, such as the study of medical ethics, coming to understand the dispute itself and the nature of each position addressed to that issue is to achieve knowledge. *Moral Issues in Health Care* achieves this by describing the major positions concerning certain moral issues and the principal objections to them. The reader should be aware, however, that I do not always maintain neutrality; in places, I endorse certain positions unequivocally. It goes without saying that it is not necessary for the reader to agree with the conclusions that I support in order to learn from this book.

Seven of the eight chapters in this book deal with substantive moral problems in the field of medical ethics. The remaining chapter, the first, is devoted to a more abstract controversy in ethical theory, which must be dealt with before particular moral problems are discussed. The issue addressed there is whether ethical disputes are the sort to which there are correct answers. Many students enter a course in ethics believing (or thinking they believe) in what might be called subjectivism or relativism. They claim that in moral matters there are no right or wrong answers. Until this issue is resolved, any discussion of particular moral problems will, at best, seem premature. Chapter 2 focuses on two questions that medical practitioners must often face: (1) whether it is ever appropriate to breach the confidence of patients and (2) whether patients should always be told the truth about their condition. Chapter 3 discusses paternalism in medicine, in particular whether it is ever permissible to treat patients without their consent. Subsequent chapters are devoted to the use of human beings as experimental subjects, euthanasia, abortion, the right to health care, unionization for medical workers, and the acquisition and distribution of scarce medical resources. The "Suggestions for

Further Reading" at the end of each chapter list more advanced readings on the topics in question. The Appendix includes eight codes of medical ethics.

In developing a work such as this, one incurs many debts. Cheryl Amason typed the entire second draft of this manuscript; for her able assistance I am most grateful.

Intellectual debts are more difficult to acknowledge. As I wrote about certain positions, arguments, and objections, I realized that I had encountered some of the ideas previously. On some occasions, however, I was unable to remember whether the source was a book or article, a discussion with another philosopher, or a suggestion by a student. I do remember my main sources of information for the discussion in Chapter 1, though. Most of the material presented there was inspired (long ago) by the lectures of, and discussions with, Norman Dahl and Barry Hoffmaster. I should point out, however, that changes and additions have been made and I am fully responsible for any errors that might remain.

Several anonymous referees provided extensive reports on the first draft of this manuscript. Their comments forced me to clarify, rethink, and revise many of the points that I made, and I am happy to thank them for their contribution.

A special thanks is owed to Marilyn Lee McConnell for her expert advice on medical matters and for her patience and encouragement.

Terrance C. McConnell

# Contents

# 1

# Ethical Theory

Ethics or ethical theory is a study of moral beliefs. After briefly indicating the various ways in which moral beliefs can be examined, this chapter will focus on one fundamental question: Can moral disputes be resolved rationally? That is, are there uniquely correct answers to moral questions or is it possible that each of several disputants is correct? If a person is convinced that there are correct answers to moral questions, it will be important to examine theories that purport to provide such answers. At the conclusion of this chapter several normative theories that are of particular interest in medical ethics will be examined.

## THE STUDY OF ETHICS

There are at least three different ways to study moral beliefs. The first way might be called *descriptive ethics*. Here a person is merely concerned with stating what the *actual* moral beliefs of some person or group of persons are. This is the sort of question that interests anthropologists, sociologists, and historians. The activity in this case is an empirical one; the idea is simply to describe what certain people *think* is right or wrong. No evaluation of these beliefs takes place. Thus, if an instructor were to distribute a survey to the class members asking about their views on abortion, euthanasia, and capital punishment, and then compile the results, this would be an example of descriptive ethics. Falling within the province of the social sciences, philosophy is not concerned with descriptive ethics as such.

*Normative ethics* comprises the second way to study moral beliefs. Here a person is concerned not merely with what someone thinks is right, but with what *really* is right. The focus of normative ethics is not in stating someone's moral beliefs; rather the interest lies in the *justification* that can be given to support those beliefs. Thus normative ethics

1

would ask whether abortion is ever permissible, if so under what conditions, and what sort of reasons or arguments can be given to support these claims. Normative ethics also asks the following: What is it that right actions have in common? What makes an action right? Why is breaking a promise wrong, but helping a person in need right? Clearly philosophers and all persons interested in medical ethics should be concerned with questions of this sort.

*Analytical ethics* is the *third* way to study moral beliefs. Here questions are asked about ethics itself. By stepping back, as it were, to ask what occurs when people discuss moral questions, the meaning of terms like "right," "wrong," "good," and "bad" is investigated. When people argue about moral matters—for example, the issue of mercy killing—can those disputes be rationally settled? This also is an area of study with which philosophers are concerned.

Our study of medical ethics will be primarily an exercise in normative ethics. We will be asking such questions as: Should a physician or a nurse tell a dying patient the truth about his or her condition? Is it ever permissible for a medical worker to breach the confidence of his or her patient? And most importantly, we will be interested in the kinds of reasons or arguments that can be given to support particular answers to these questions. For the most part, we will not be interested in descriptive ethics. There is an exception to this, however. On some occasions we will examine briefly the various codes of medical ethics, such as the Hippocratic Oath and the AMA Principles of Medical Ethics. The purpose of this will be to see what certain members of the medical community have thought about some of these issues.

## SUBJECTIVISM AND OBJECTIVISM

But before embarking on this fascinating journey in normative ethics, the most fundamental question raised in the area of analytical ethics must be asked. If we do not come to terms with this question, the whole journey may seem pointless. The question concerns the nature of moral judgments. Are moral judgments subjective or objective? When a discipline or area of inquiry is *objective*, there are correct and incorrect answers to questions in that area. By contrast, when a discipline or area of inquiry is *subjective*, questions in that area do not admit of correct or incorrect answers. It is commonly said that if an area is subjective, then assertions in that area are *just a matter of opinion*. An area that presumably everyone would agree is subjective is taste in ice cream. If one person says that chocolate ice cream is good and another says that it is not good, it is not thought that one person is correct and the other wrong. Rather it is thought that taste in ice cream is just a matter of opinion. On the other hand, disciplines such as chemistry, physics, and history are ones that most people think are objective. Thus if two people disagree about the percentage of a certain chemical in a given solution, one of them must be wrong. Similarly, if two people disagree about whether George Washington really died on a certain date, at least one of them is mistaken.

This explanation enables us to give more precise definitions of the terms "objective" and "subjective." Moral judgments, such as "act A is right (wrong)," are *objective* just in case for any two people, if one person affirms the judgment "A is right" and the other denies it, at least one of them is mistaken. On the other hand, moral judgments, such as "act A is right (wrong)," are *subjective* just in case it is possible for there to be two people such that one affirms "A is right" and the other denies it, and neither of them need be mistaken. Thus, concerning a debate about abortion, the subjectivist might say the following. Person $P_1$ thinks that abortion is always wrong, and person $P_2$ thinks that abortions are right if that is what the woman really wants. Neither $P_1$ nor $P_2$ is incorrect. It is all a matter of opinion. Abortion is wrong for $P_1$ but right for $P_2$. The objectivist, by contrast, will say that the moral belief of at least one of those persons is mistaken. Notice, by the way, that the definitions proposed here, if adapted to the discipline in question, capture our judgments about the examples presented earlier. Clearly the issue of whether chocolate ice cream is really good is subjective; two people can disagree about that matter and neither need be mistaken. But this is not the case when we ask about the percentage of a certain chemical in a given solution, or when we discuss the date on which George Washington died.

Many people are subjectivists, or at least think that they are. But many claim to be subjectivists for bad reasons, misunderstanding objectivism. In other words, many people oppose objectivism because they reject certain theses that they assume the objectivist must hold, when in fact he or she need not. To illustrate, let us examine a position called *absolutism*. Absolutism is the view that all moral rules hold necessarily and without exception. For example, someone might say that the essence of morality consists in the Ten Commandments, and that everyone must obey each of these rules without exception. Or outside of a religious context, someone might say that the usual prohibitions against killing, stealing, and breaking promises all hold without exception. Many people deny that moral judgments are objective because they reject absolutism; they think that there are legitimate exceptions to most moral rules. However, one who holds that moral judgments are objective need not say that absolutism is true. The objectivist is only committed to saying that one general moral principle holds without exception. This can be illustrated if the notion that contrasts with absolutism is explained, the idea that moral judgments are *context-dependent*. A moral judgment is context-dependent if the same kind of action (or action-type) can be right in one context (or set of circumstances) and wrong in another context (or set of circumstances). Most people reject absolutism. They believe, for example, that though a person normally ought to tell the truth, it is permissible to lie to a would-be murderer concerning the whereabouts of his or her intended victim. And though most of us believe that a person normally ought to keep a promise, it is permissible to break a promise to meet a friend for lunch in order to save the life of someone who has been in an accident.

It seems quite plausible, then, to hold that moral judgments are context-dependent. But the objectivist can allow this; the objectivist need not be an absolutist. As was stated earlier, the objectivist need only say that one moral principle holds without exception. Let us illustrate this by noting the relationship between a general moral principle and some particular moral rules. The following example of a general moral principle shall be considered: Always do that which will maximize human happiness. The following diagram shows some of the particular moral rules that might follow from this general principle.

Maximize human happiness (general principle)

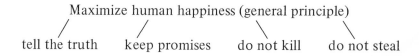

tell the truth    keep promises    do not kill    do not steal

Certainly in most cases a person would have to obey these rules in order to maximize human happiness. But extreme circumstances can be imagined which force a person to break the rules in order to effect the greatest amount of happiness. The examples given in the previous paragraph suggest cases in which someone can maximize human happiness only by not telling the truth and by breaking a promise. Similarly, a situation can be imagined in which someone must kill a person in order to prevent that person from killing others. And, as in the myth of Robin Hood, robbing from the very rich in order to feed the poor might be justified. So though these rules hold for the most part, there are exceptions to them. It is important, though, to realize that those exceptions are made on a *principled* basis, and allowing these exceptions is compatible with objectivism.

To illustrate, if the general principle (maximize human happiness) is correct, then in each situation what *really ought to be done* is that action that will maximize human happiness. And, presumably, it is an objective matter (though it may be difficult to determine in practice) which act in any given situation will maximize human happiness. This example illustrates that the objectivist can allow that moral judgments are context-dependent.

## ARGUMENTS FOR SUBJECTIVISM: A CRITICAL ASSESSMENT

If someone's reason for being a subjectivist is based upon a rejection of absolutism, these grounds are insufficient. There are, however, other reasons that people have given for being subjectivists. A critical examination of the major reasons (or arguments) given to support subjectivism follows.

The *first* reason to support subjectivism is that there is widespread disagreement on moral matters, both between and within societies. Furthermore, people rarely change their minds on moral matters; each person thinks that his or her moral views are the right ones. It is true, of course, that there is a considerable amount of disagreement with regard to moral matters. The mere fact that there is widespread disagreement, however, does not show that morality is a subjective matter. It does not follow that an area of inquiry is subjective just because people come up with conflicting answers. Objectivism with respect to any area does not entail that everyone will in fact agree about what answers are correct. Notice that there is not universal agreement in the various sciences, but few draw the inference that these areas are subjective. Physicists still do not agree whether light is a wave, a particle, or something else. At one time in the history of science astronomers could not agree if the sun or the earth was the center of our universe. And today, though many people believe that diseases are caused by viruses, some think that they are caused by demons or the gods. But we are never tempted to conclude from this that what the nature of light is, what the center of the universe is, and what the cause of disease is are all matters of opinion. The mere presence of disagreement in an area, then, does not prove that the discipline in question is subjective.

The *second* reason to support moral subjectivism is that people acquire their moral beliefs from their parents, peer groups, and their particular society. The moral beliefs a person has depends on the environment in which he or she has been raised. Moral beliefs are *not discovered*; it is rather a matter of assimilation. Moreover, since people have different environments, agreement about moral matters may never be achieved. It might first be noted, as just seen, that whether agreement in ethics is achieved is not relevant to the issue of objectivity. But there are other difficulties with this second argument. How someone acquires a belief is irrelevant to the assessment of that belief. How Einstein came upon his general theory of relativity does not affect our assessment of that theory. Similarly, then, how someone acquires moral beliefs is not relevant to the correctness or incorrectness of those beliefs. Finally, it should be noted that people acquire scientific beliefs, historical beliefs, and in fact all individual beliefs, from their environment. And if this reasoning shows that morality is subjective, it will show that all areas of inquiry are subjective, an extreme view few people are willing to adopt.

*Third*, the uncertainty of our moral judgments is often cited as another reason to support subjectivism. Moral matters seem very complicated. A woman considering an abortion, for example, might have some reason to believe that carrying the child to full term will threaten her life, but she cannot be sure that it will. And think of the loss to the world if this child would have made contributions comparable to those of Isaac Newton or Marie Curie. Making moral judgments is hopeless, and so morality is subjective. There are two things to say in response to this argument. First, it is not an argument for subjectivism at all; it could not show that moral judgments are neither correct nor incorrect. Rather, it is an argument for ethical skepticism, the view that we cannot know what the right answers to moral questions are. The argument actually presupposes that moral beliefs are correct or incorrect. Second, if certainty were the criterion that we used to determine what fields are objective, few if any disciplines would pass the test of objectivity. The physical sciences would not be objective; nor would history. Judgments in each of these areas are constantly being revised. At most, logic and mathematics would satisfy this criterion. Making certainty a necessary condition of objectivity, then, is much too strict. Areas of inquiry that most want to say are objective would fail this test, and so this reason does not show that moral judgments are subjective.

*Fourth*, it is often said that there are no moral authorities, no moral experts. Some even suggest that the very notion of moral expertise is an absurdity. This idea is sometimes expressed when people ask, "Who are you to say what is right?" This argument gains additional credibility when the presence of experts in other areas is noted; for example, there are experts in the various branches of the physical sciences. So if morality were objective, there should be experts in that field too. Since there are no moral experts, grounds exist for believing that morality is subjective. This is an important argument that many have found convincing. There are, however, several critical responses that can be made to it. First, the objectivist might agree that there are no moral experts, but claim that this does not establish subjectivism. The objectivist need not say that anyone *knows* what should be done in a given situation. The objectivist is only committed to saying that there *is* a correct answer. Of course, since there are experts in other areas believed to be objective, the objectivist owes us an explanation as to why there are no moral experts. The objectivist might say that ethics is a very difficult field; there is still no established body of knowledge in the area of morality, and thus there are no experts.

Few, however, have been satisfied with this explanation. People have been grappling with moral questions long before the days of Socrates, and so it is reasonable to expect that some progress in the field would have been made. If the objectivist agrees that there are no moral experts, he or she would be well-advised to search for a different explanation of that fact.

A second response to the "no moral experts" argument is this. The objectivist can point out that among the disputants there are not authorities in the other disciplines either. When two physicists argue about a certain matter, they do not appeal to some "super" physicist to settle the dispute; similarly, neither chemists nor historians settle disputes in this manner. The physicist, chemist, and historian play the role of the expert vis-à-vis the layman. And it happens that since all people are moral agents, no one is a layman in ethics. A person can avoid the sciences, but being a moral agent is impossible to avoid.

The third response to the argument, though, is the one that most objectivists will probably favor. The objectivist can claim that there are in fact moral experts, namely, moral philosophers. The subjectivist, of course, is likely to challenge that claim by asking why moral philosophers do not offer ready answers to particular problems in their area. As most people know, those who go to moral philosophers with difficult ethical problems rarely get straightforward, unequivocal advice. But if someone has a problem in any of the physical sciences, a satisfactory answer is likely if the problem is taken to an expert. The objectivist can answer this important challenge, however, by pointing out that knowledge of what should be done in a particular situation depends on both knowledge of general moral principles and of the facts of the particular situation. The moral expert will have the former knowledge, of course, but there is no reason to believe that he or she will be an expert with regard to factual matters. To illustrate, consider this simple example: A moral expert may advise a couple that they should not have a child if the risks that the child will be severely deformed are great. In so counseling the couple, the moral expert is appealing to a general moral principle. But unless the moral expert also happens to be an authority in genetics, he or she cannot tell this particular couple whether any child they have will be deformed. This is why moral experts are unable to give quick and simple answers to ethical problems. There are, then, three responses to show that the "no moral experts" argument for subjectivism fails.

*Fifth*, the most popular argument embraced by beginning students of ethics in defense of subjectivism is that it is the more plausible position because bad consequences ensue if a person adopts objectivism. In particular, it is claimed that objectivists are *dogmatic* and *intolerant*. And, it is argued, open-mindedness and tolerance follow from the adoption of subjectivism. Thus subjectivism is preferred.

Whatever initial appeal this argument might have, its underlying reasoning is surely confused. First, neither open-mindedness nor tolerance follows from subjectivism. To be open-minded is to be willing to change one's moral views in light of the criticisms of others. But subjectivists have no reason to alter their moral views because they say that moral views are neither correct nor incorrect. A person cannot take criticism seriously if his or her views cannot be incorrect. And why should the subjectivist be tolerant of the moral opinions of others? Nothing in the subjectivist's doctrine suggests an obligation to respect the views of others. Clearly, the subjectivist's ground for respecting the moral views of others cannot be that those views might be correct; according to the subjectivist, no views are correct. Second, if it followed from subjectivism that the moral agent ought to be open-minded and tolerant, then subjectivism would be self-refuting. If the moral agent *ought* to be tolerant, then at least one moral judgment is correct, contrary to subjectivism. Finally, an objectivist need be neither dogmatic nor intolerant. The objectivist says that there are right and wrong answers to moral questions, not that such answers are known. Moreover, if an objectivist is consistent, open-mindedness is necessary. If someone says that there are correct and incorrect answers in a given discipline, then that person must admit that it is logically possible that his or her answers are wrong. Of course, not all objectivists are open-minded. But this is not a problem with the position of objectivism; rather the problem is that the *people* who adopt objectivism are sometimes inconsistent.

It is sometimes argued that one cannot prove or disprove moral judgments in the way that scientific judgments are proved or disproved.

This is the *sixth* reason to support subjectivism. To respond fully to this subjectivist argument is not possible here. The argument does raise several important questions, however. Are moral judgments different from scientific ones? If so, how? And, are they different in such a way that leads to the (justifiable) belief that objectivism holds in the sciences but not in ethics? The answers to these questions are not obvious. Nevertheless, there are two ways that the objectivist can respond. First, the objectivist can point out that if a certain theory about the nature of moral judgments is correct, a theory called naturalism, then ethical statements can be verified or justified in exactly the same way that scientific ones are. (Naturalism is the view that moral judgments are disguised empirical statements.) Of course, for this answer to be totally convincing, the objectivist must provide a full-blown defense of naturalism. Second, the objectivist might argue that when one has two different fields of inquiry, such as ethics and science, there may well be two different canons of rationality for establishing and justifying beliefs within those fields. Individuals have a right to question the objectivist about the nature of this different method for settling ethical disputes, of course, but this is a reasonable move for the objectivist to make.

## ARGUMENTS FOR OBJECTIVISM

The usual reasons given to support subjectivism are not sufficient. But this argument by criticism does not prove that objectivism itself is correct. If positive arguments to support objectivism cannot be provided, judgment on this issue can be withheld. Several positive arguments will be presented here. These arguments are designed to show that most people really believe that moral judgments are objective. The first argument, (A1), may be stated as follows.

(A1) 1. Moral disputes do occur, situations in which each disputant is trying to convince the other to adopt his or her positon on the moral question at issue.

2. When moral disputes occur, we (either participants or spectators) do not ordinarily regard the activity as silly or irrational. On the contrary, we normally regard the activity as quite serious.

3. But if we believed that subjectivism were true, then we would regard moral disputes as silly or irrational.

4. Therefore subjectivism conflicts with one of our basic beliefs about the moral life.

Argument (A1) will be convincing only if each of the premises is plausible. Premises (1) and (2) are surely correct and need no defense. But why should one accept (3)? It seems that a subjectivist must say that moral disputes (not rooted in factual disagreement) are silly or irrational. It makes no sense for two people to argue about a matter to which there can, in principle, be no correct answer. Notice how we would regard a dispute about whether a certain flavor of ice cream is really good, a matter that is clearly subjective. Since this question is not subject to rational resolution, debating it is pointless. And it should be clear that the objectivist *can* explain why moral disputes (not rooted in factual disagreement) are neither silly nor irrational: the disputants are seeking the correct answer to an important question.

The subjectivist may still insist that (3) is false. To defend this claim, the subjectivist might argue that moral disputes, unlike debates about the goodness of a certain flavor of ice cream, have important consequences for the losers. People *act* on their moral beliefs, and their actions affect others. Suppose, for example, that my society is considering whether to institute capital punishment and I am opposed to such a practice. If I lose this debate, if my society adopts capital punishment, this can have an adverse effect on my interests. It certainly will if I am convicted of a capital offense. In this case when others act on a moral belief which I do not hold, I will be harmed. The same will be true if I take a person's privacy to be an important right while others put no value on this. Thus, the subjectivist argues, moral disputes make sense, not because there are right answers to such questions, but rather because one must protect one's interests. This response shows that the subjectivist can account for why some moral disputes are regarded as neither silly nor irrational. But by no means does this explanation fit all cases. Those who oppose a moral belief even though they do not believe that their loved ones will be harmed if others act on that belief are behaving irrationally, according to this view. It follows, then, that if someone opposes voluntary euthansia, not because that person believes that bad consequences will ensue from its adoption (and hence potential harm to oneself), but rather because of the nature of the act, the person is behaving irrationally. The same must be said of a person who opposes abortion for only those who want it, or of a person who regards prostitution as wrong (again, when the basis for these judgments is not the belief that bad consequences will follow from such acts). In neither case does the person regard his or her interests as being threatened. But surely such a conclusion is too extreme. Even if we regard those who oppose voluntary euthanasia, abortion on request, and prostitution as morally mistaken, we surely do not think that the very act of arguing against these practices is irrational. Hence premise (3), properly qualified, is true.

It might be objected that argument (A1) merely shows that we do not *believe* that subjectivism is true; and since this belief might be false, we do not have a strict proof of objectivism. This, of course, is correct. But it does not mean that argument (A1) is unimportant. (A1) is an argument designed to shift the burden of proof. It shows how radically at odds with our ordinary beliefs about the moral life subjectivism is. Since any adequate metaethical theory must be in accord with fundamental beliefs about the moral life and the common use of moral terms, considerable doubt has been cast on subjectivism. At the very least the onus is on the subjectivist to show why the ordinary view of moral disputes is mistaken.

A second argument to support objectivism appeals to the way people regard the behavior of moral agents facing predicaments or difficult moral problems.

(A2) 1. Moral predicaments do occur, situations in which the agent believes that there are reasons for doing each of two actions both of which cannot be done, and the agent does not know which is the more important.
2. When an agent is in a moral predicament, moral advice is often sought.
3. That agents seek advice in such situations seems appropriate, and certainly not irrational.
4. But if subjectivism were believed to be true, seeking moral advice would be regarded as inappropriate and irrational.
5. Therefore subjectivism conflicts with a basic belief about the moral life.

Again, this argument will render the conclusion plausible only if the premises can be defended. The first three premises are uncontroversial and cannot seriously be questioned. But is premise (4) correct? It seems that it is. If an agent can examine all of the facts, then according to subjectivism there is nothing to seek advice about. Since the subjectivist says that answers to moral questions are neither correct nor incorrect (or are not subject to rational assessment), the subjectivist must regard seeking advice about ethical matters as being on a par with asking someone else what flavor of ice cream is really good. Such behavior must be looked on as pointless and irrational because nothing that the person says can help one make a better or more rational moral decision.

The subjectivist will undoubtedly want to reject (4), and will do so by arguing that it is not silly, inappropriate, or irrational to consult with people about moral matters because acting on moral beliefs has serious consequences. People must come to an understanding with each other about moral beliefs in order to avoid terrible consequences. Note, for example, how chaotic and miserable life would be if people did not generally agree that stealing is wrong. Thus, even though moral questions cannot be rationally resolved, it makes sense to seek advice and consult about such matters; doing so promotes social stability. Again, however, this response applies to only some moral disputes. There are many situations in which a person appropriately seeks advice, though the subjectivist's explanation is inapplicable. The issue of suicide provides an example. The consequences need not be disastrous if there is no general agreement among members of our society concerning this question. Yet we certainly think that a person contemplating suicide is behaving quite appropriately if that person seeks advice before acting. And his or her behavior is not less appropriate if there are no relatives who might suffer or be harmed by a successful suicide. It seems, then, that the subjectivist must say that seeking advice in situations like this is irrational. Such a conclusion, however, is not plausible. So, in spite of the subjectivist's objection, premise (4) of (A2) holds true for a large number of cases, and that is all the objectivist needs.

A third argument for objectivism appeals to the way that agents behave after they have faced a difficult moral situation, and it may be sketched as follows.

(A3) 1. People sometimes experience moral doubt after they have acted.
2. That moral doubt occurs seems appropriate, and certainly not irrational.
3. But if we believed that subjectivism were true, experiencing moral doubt would normally be regarded as inappropriate or irrational.
4. Therefore subjectivism conflicts with a basic belief about the moral life.

The first two premises of this argument are self-explanatory and surely quite plausible. Premise (3), however, requires a brief explanation. Under normal circumstances experiencing moral doubt must be regarded by the subjectivist as irrational; an individual cannot sensibly doubt whether what he or she did was really right or wrong when, by hypothesis, no actions are really right or wrong. Doubt is a rational attitude only if the individual can be mistaken, and the subjectivist is committed to saying that there can be no such thing as a purely moral mistake. The subjectivist might retort that the reason that doubt about moral matters is appropriate is that the individual is worried about the practical consequences of being assessed negatively by society. This retaliation may take the form of moral censure, or something more severe, such as incarceration. That doubt is regarded as appropriate, then, does not commit us to objectivism. However plausible this response may seem, it cannot begin to explain adequately all cases. Having had an abortion, a woman may seriously question whether she has done the right thing even though she believes that no one else will find out about this act. The source of her worry is not that she will be blamed by her society, yet we certainly do not regard her doubt as irrational. This and similar examples show that premise (3) of argument (A3) is true of a number of cases and that the subjectivist's response is inadequate.

Let us consider one other argument to support objectivism.

(A4) 1. If we believed that subjectivism were true, then the only way that we could legitimately criticize someone else's moral views would be to show that they are internally inconsistent.

2. So if we believe subjectivism is true, we cannot criticize the moral views of someone like Hitler (assuming that his views are consistent).

3. But we do want to say that there is something wrong with Hitler's moral views, even if (and perhaps especially if) they are consistent.

4. So we cannot accept the consequences of subjectivism.

A word of explanation concerning premise (1) is in order. A subjectivist can criticize the moral views of another even if he or she believes that those views are consistent. But the subjectivist cannot regard himself or herself as trying to show that those views are mistaken. Morality is not the sort of thing about which one can be mistaken, according to the subjectivist. Rather the subjectivist must regard himself or herself as being engaged in a propaganda effort. In criticizing someone's views on an ethical matter, we are not trying to show that the person is wrong; we are simply trying to convince others to adopt our favorite view. But is that what we are really doing when we criticize the moral views of a racist like Hitler? A rigorous subjectivist may be willing to say this. But for most of us, it is not a viable alternative. These four arguments show how fundamentally subjectivism conflicts with widely held beliefs about the moral life. Although it is possible that such beliefs are incorrect, the burden of proof remains on the subjectivist. Unless the subjectivist can respond, there are good reasons for holding that moral judgments are objective.

## MORAL THEORIES

If moral judgments are objective—if there are right and wrong answers to moral questions—then knowledge of the criteria of rightness and wrongness is desirable. What characteristics make an action right? There are, as might be expected, different theories regarding this question. This chapter discusses only the two most general theories about what makes an action right; further intricacies involved in these theories will not be dealt with. As it happens, the conflict between these two types of theories emerges in our examination of most of the particular moral problems that constitute the field that we call medical ethics. It is important, then, to understand the basic differences between these two theories.

### Consequentialism

Consequentialist moral theories (sometimes called teleological) hold that the rightness or wrongness of actions is determined solely by the value of the consequences those actions produce. The inherent nature of the action is not relevant to whether it is right or wrong. The only thing that counts in assessing the action is the value of the consequences. Consequentialists assent to the familiar maxim that the end justifies the means. According to consequentialism, then, an act is right if and only if it produces consequences at least as good as the consequences of any alternative act open to the agent. Consequentialist theories are alike in that they require an agent to maximize the good; they differ with respect to whose good it is that the agent must maximize. One consequentialist theory not to be discussed is ethical egoism, the view that an agent ought to maximize personal interests only. The most popular consequentialist theory, though, and the one that will be of greatest interest to us in our discussion of the basic issues of medical ethics, is *utilitarianism*. Utilitarianism requires an agent to do that action which brings about the greatest balance of good over evil in the universe as a whole; that is, utilitarianism requires an agent to maximize the good of all humans or, as some utilitarians prefer, of all sentient beings. Whenever someone is about to act, that person must consider all of the available alternatives and perform that act which will maximize the good of all affected parties.

Egoism and utilitarianism are not the only possibilities, however; one other version of consequentialism is worth noting. *Patient consequentialism* requires a person to maximize the good of a selected group. This is a consequentialist theory that might be adopted by medical workers. Like utilitarianism, this view judges the rightness or wrongness of an act by looking only at the consequences. But unlike utilitarianism, patient consequentialism instructs a medical worker to bring about the greatest balance of good over evil for a particular group of persons, namely, his or her patients. Thus medical workers are required to do whatever is best for patients. Certainly many physicians and nurses preach patient consequentialism; whether they practice it, or whether they should practice it, however, is another matter.

## Deontologism

Not everyone agrees with the moral outlook of the consequentialist. The views of nonconsequentialists are usually called *deontological moral theories*. Put simply, the deontologist denies what the consequentialist affirms; that is, the moral status of an action is *not* determined *solely* by the consequences. What else could be relevant to assessing an action? According to the deontologist the *kind* or *type* of action an agent performs is also morally relevant; the inherent nature of an action, as well as the consequences it produces, can make a moral difference. Consequentialists are concerned only with what happens or what state of affairs is produced. As long as the greatest good or the least amount of evil is produced, it does not matter who the agents were or what sort of acts they performed. By contrast, deontologists are usually concerned not only with what happens, but also with what people do; the nature of the act is morally important. For example, the deontologist might hold that if an action is one of killing an innocent person, that is morally decisive against the act even if it would produce very good consequences. Or the deontologist might hold that if an action is one of torturing another human being, that counts against the action regardless of how good the consequences of doing that act in a particular situation might be. Or again, if an action is one of knowingly punishing an innocent person, the deontologist might hold that the act is wrong regardless of the goodness of the consequences. The deontologist, then, denies that the end justifies the means.

Generally, deontologists and utilitarians differ with respect to the status they assign to moral rules. For the utilitarian, moral rules are merely *rules of thumb*. They are useful in telling one what actions are generally right, but there are always exceptions to moral rules. An agent must consider each situation anew in making moral decisions. Usually such actions as lying, stealing, and killing will not maximize the good of all affected parties. But if in some particular case one must perform such an act in order to maximize the good, then utilitarianism entails that one is obligated to do so. The deontologist, by contrast, tends to take moral rules more seriously. Moral rules forbidding such heinous acts as killing and torturing are ones which may rarely, if ever, be broken. As we shall see, when we discuss the issues of confidentiality and truth-telling, one of the important questions concerns the status of moral rules.

To clarify the difference between consequentialist and deontological moral theories, consider the following. Suppose that a moral assessment of the decision of President Truman to drop the atomic bomb on Hiroshima is being made. The only factors that a consequentialist will consider in assessing this action will be its consequences. How did the consequences of this act compare with those of the available alternatives? Examining the case superficially, it might be said that some of the important consequences were these: the destruction of thousands of human lives; the production of genetic deformities in the offspring of some of the survivors; the saving of X number of lives because the act ended the war Y years earlier than it would have ended had the act not been performed; etc. The consequentialist must look at all of these consequences and "weigh them up," as it were. Clearly the act of dropping the bomb caused some bad consequences. But perhaps these bad consequences were outweighed by the good ones; perhaps in this terrible situation that was the best of the available alternatives open to the President. The deontologist will go about assessing the act in a very different way. The deontologist might say that the act of killing thousands of innocent human beings is wrong, regardless of the consequences; or it might be said that the act of saving one's country is the right thing for a chief executive to do. Since Truman's act can be described accurately in many different ways, deontologists are apt to disagree among themselves concerning its assessment. But whatever judgment the deontologist reaches, reasons will be cited to justify the judgment that are different from those appealed to by the consequentialist.

## MORAL PROBLEMS

Throughout this book particular moral problems will be examined. It will be noted how utilitarian considerations are often cited to support a certain position and how deontological considerations are appealed to in defending a competing view. Since our task is to examine some of the moral problems in medicine, let us be clear about what is meant. A *moral problem*, as the term is used here, is a situation in which there are moral considerations to support one action, say act $A$, yet there are moral considerations to support another action, act $B$. Act $A$ and act $B$ cannot both be done, but it must be known which is more important morally—which is the right act. When what ought to be done is not known, a state of moral perplexity prevails.

An assumption that will be made throughout this book should be stated at the outset. Some people believe that many of the moral problems encountered in medical contexts are ones for which uniquely correct answers cannot be provided. It is not the subjectivist who is being referred to here. Rather this is a person who says that there are *genuine moral dilemmas* and that many of the moral problems in medical contexts are genuinely dilemmatic. A genuine moral dilemma is a situation in which a person really ought (all things considered) to do each of two things, both of which cannot be done. No matter what the person does, he or she will do something wrong (or will fail to do something that ought to be done). An agent in a genuine dilemma is, in a sense, morally doomed. Moral dilemmas are *irresolvable* moral problems. No further moral work will help an agent in these situations.

In discussing ethical questions in the ensuing chapters, it will be assumed that there are no genuine moral dilemmas.[1] There are, of course, moral problems. Many of these moral problems are agonizing. What is being assumed here is that these problems have solutions. These solutions are difficult to establish; they often require a great expenditure of intellectual energy. Unless there are, at least in principle, solutions to these conflicts, further investigation is superfluous. Our discussion, then, will proceed on the assumption that there are uniquely correct solutions to the moral problems that arise in medical contexts.

## SUMMARY

The principal focus of this chapter has been on the dispute between the subjectivist and the objectivist, a dispute about the most fundamental issue in analytical ethics. Arguments for each of the positions were examined. The arguments supporting subjectivism appear seriously flawed. And while the arguments to support objectivism are not logically conclusive, they do shift the burden of proof; they show that the tenets of objectivism better fit our beliefs about the moral life. Toward the end of the chapter our focus shifted to normative theories. The difference between consequentialist and deontological theories was examined. It was noted that while there are several forms of consequentialist theories, in the context of medical ethics two theories are of particular interest: utilitarianism and patient consequentialism. As we examine particular moral issues that arise in the delivery of health care, we shall see that deontological and consequentialist considerations will often emerge as competitors.

## CASE STUDY

Suppose that a Nazi war criminal responsible for the cruel torture and deaths of many innocent people escaped in 1945. He was a high ranking officer in the Nazi army, so it was deemed important to capture and punish him. The pursuit of him, however, was unsuccessful. For the past 30 years he has been living *incognito* in a South American village. He has become a useful and prosperous member of the community; indeed, he has been a model citizen. In 1980, because of the work of an investigative reporter, the identity and whereabouts of this war criminal, now 70 years old, are made known.[2]

### Discussion Questions

1. Should the Nazi war criminal be punished? Why?
2. If he should be punished, what type of punishment would be appropriate?
3. Consider the reasons that might be given to support the claim that he should not be punished. Are there considerations consequentialist or deontological in nature?
4. Consider the reasons that might be given to support the claim that he should be punished. Are these considerations consequentialist or deontological in nature?

## SUGGESTIONS FOR FURTHER READING

William K. Frankena, *Ethics*, Second Edition (Englewood Cliffs, New Jersey: Prentice-Hall, 1973), pp. 1–9 and 12–43.
Gilbert Harman, *The Nature of Morality* (New York: Oxford University Press, 1977), pp. 3–52 and 91–99.
John Ladd (ed.), *Relativism* (Belmont, Calif.: Wadsworth Publishing Co., 1973).

J.L. Mackie, *Ethics: Inventing Right and Wrong* (New York: Penguin Books, 1977), pp. 15-49.

Paul W. Taylor, *Principles of Ethics* (Belmont, Calif.: Dickenson Publishing Co., 1975), pp. 1-29.

## NOTES

1. The assumption that there are no genuine moral dilemmas is defended in my paper, "Moral Dilemmas and Consistency in Ethics," *Canadian Journal of Philosophy*, Vol. VIII (1978), pp. 269-287.
2. This type of case is discussed by R.S. Downie, "The Justification of Punishment," in James Rachels (ed.), *Moral Problems* (New York: Harper & Row, 1971), pp. 223-224.

# 2

# Moral Problems in the Medical Worker-Patient Relationship

After some introductory remarks about understanding the nature of and being able to identify moral problems in medical contexts, our focus shall turn to several ethical issues that arise in the context of the one-to-one relationship between the medical worker and the patient. One general issue concerns the way in which the relationship between the medical worker and the patient should be conceived. Different models of that relationship will be discussed and the moral differences among these models will be highlighted. Two particular moral problems will then be discussed. The first concerns the confidentiality of communications between the patient and the medical worker. Are there any conditions under which the medical worker may breach this confidence? If so, when? The second concerns telling the patient the truth about his or her condition. Is it ever permissible for a medical worker to withhold the truth from the patient about his or her condition? If so, when?

## IDENTIFYING MORAL PROBLEMS

As one physician has remarked, the issues discussed in medical ethics have changed radically in the past twenty-five years.[1] In what now seems the distant past the issues of medical ethics included the following: How large should the physician's sign be? Should the physician prescribe over the telephone? Should the physician split fees with persons referring patients? Should the physician's specialty be listed after his or her name in the Yellow Pages? Some of these questions may still be of some interest and importance, but by and large the contemporary questions to which medical ethics is addressed seem much more serious. Euthanasia and abortion, genetic engineering, and issues concerned with the distribution of medical care, such as the right to health care and the allocation of scarce medical resources, are several of these topics. In some respects this shift in the questions and issues discussed is a symptom of the success of medicine. Now that patients can be kept alive for an indefinite period through the use of respirators, intravenous feeding, and the like, the question of whether it is always appropriate to do so must be faced. This presents a challenge to a value judgment that was unquestioned in medical fields in the past: life, the highest value, is worth preserving at any cost. Advances in the field of genetics have led to new moral problems concerning the use to which that knowledge is put. To what extent should scientists engage in genetic engineering? Is it appropriate to "modify man"?

It is important for us to be able to distinguish moral problems from other sorts of problems that arise in medical contexts. To see how confusions might arise, consider the following three cases.[2]

## CASE 1

Dr. A's hospital has only one unit of a rare piece of medical equipment. A person with a terminal illness who will die soon is presently using that machinery. A young accident victim arrives at the hospital. This person's life can be saved by using the special equipment; without it, however, this person will die. Dr. A believes that he has a moral obligation to remove the equipment from the terminally ill patient and to allow the accident victim to use it. The terminally ill patient, however, is Dr. A's wife and he cannot muster up the strength to remove her from the machinery.

## CASE 2

Dr. B is dedicated to her profession. She believes that she is morally obligated to do the best that she can for each patient. A man with two serious medical problems, a brain tumor and a weak heart, comes to Dr. B for help. After examining the man, she cannot decide what course of action to take. If she operates on the tumor, she will probably correct that problem but at a great risk to the patient's heart. On the other hand, she may try to treat the tumor with a new form of therapy. To do so involves less danger to the heart, but the efficacy of the treatment is not known. Dr. B is not sure what to do.

## CASE 3

A woman in an isolated, rural community comes to see Dr. C. She wishes to have an abortion. Dr. C is the only physician in the area and the woman cannot afford to travel to the distant, larger cities. After examining the woman, Dr. C concludes that it would be medically safe to perform the abortion. He also believes that the laws in his state are vague enough that he can justify the act legally. Dr. C, however, has moral reservations about performing the act. He is not opposed to all abortions. But in this case he thinks that the woman's reasons for wanting to terminate the pregnancy are not good ones. Dr. C, however, is a tolerant person and believes that physicians should not impose their moral views on patients. Moreover, he realizes that if he does not perform the abortion, then the woman will be forced to have the child. Dr. C therefore wonders whether, because of the special circumstances, he should participate in an action that he otherwise believes is wrong.

These cases can be used to distinguish between moral problems and other difficulties that medical practitioners face. Recall that a moral problem is a situation in which a person has grounds for believing that there are moral reasons to support each of two courses of action, both cannot be done, and one does not know which is more important morally. Case 1 is not a moral problem (in this sense of the term). Dr. A is convinced that he does know what he ought to do. He believes that he ought to disconnect his wife from the life-prolonging equipment and make it available to the young accident victim, but he finds it very difficult—and perhaps impossible—to do this. This is a case of *moral weakness*, and its experience is common. But since Dr. A believes that he knows what he ought to do, his problem is not a moral problem.

Case 2 is also not a moral problem. In this case Dr. B is unsure what to do, but her perplexity is technical, not moral. The doctor assumes that she is obliged to provide the best medical care that she can. She is simply unsure what the best medical care is in this situation. Technical problems, of course, are quite common in medical contexts.

Case 3 is a moral problem, a kind of ethical problem that the medical practitioner must often face. In this situation Dr. C does not know what should be done. His perplexity is not legal; he knows that the law permits him to perform the abortion. And his doubts are not medical; he knows that the procedure in this case is safe. But he does not know what the right thing to do in this situation is. He thinks that the woman would be wrong to have the abortion, and so there are moral considerations that lead him to refuse to perform the operation. But he wonders whether it is appropriate for a physician to refuse to treat a patient because the physician disapproves of the treatment on moral grounds. Thus Dr. C has a moral problem.

A classic example of a moral problem—and one outside the medical field—is presented by Jean-Paul Sartre in his essay *Existentialism and Human Emotions.*[3] This problem is set in France during World War II. Sartre's student seeks his advice on the following matter. He believes that he ought to join the Free French Forces in order to contribute to the cause of defeating the German invaders. He especially feels the force of this obligation since his brother has been killed in a German offensive. On the other hand, he believes that he ought to stay with his elderly mother since he is her only source of companionship and comfort. Were he to leave her, she would become very unhappy and perhaps even die. The student is forced to make a moral choice: is his greater obligation owed to his country or to his mother?

One other point concerning moral problems is that they are virtually unavoidable. Many moral problems that an agent faces arise, not because of some wrong act that the agent performs but simply because of the nature of the world. This is certainly true of moral problems that arise in medical contexts. An excellent example to illustrate this point is presented by Robert M. Veatch.[4]

## CASE 4

A four-day-old infant was currently on a respirator suffering from respiratory deficiency that was presumably, but not definitely, related to a diagnosis of trisomy-18, a genetic defect which for unknown reasons causes gross congenital malfunctions. A clinical conference was being held in an attempt to decide what should be done in the case. The participants were the chief pediatrician, a psychiatrist, a social worker, a nurse, and a pediatrics resident.

Trisomy-18, the presence of an extra E chromosome, results in moderate to severe mental retardation, intrauterine growth failure, hypertonicity, anatomical malformations, particularly of the ears and fingers, cardiac and renal anomalies, rigidity of the body, and variable brain deformities. Fifty percent of all cases result in death in the first two months; 13 percent live more than a year. There are reports of children reaching three and ten years of age and one report of three patients, all women, reaching adulthood.

The chief of pediatrics at the hospital reported at the conference that he had held several agonizing conversations with the father of the child, who had told him, "If you cannot guarantee my child will be normal, I don't want you to do anything for it." The chief of pediatrics, who was directly responsible for this case because of the nature of the medical and moral syndrome, shared the sympathies of the father. He reported having told the father, "I promise you that I will do everything in my power to see that your wishes are fulfilled."

The psychiatric consultant reported that he had also spent considerable time with the father. He said that he thought the father was in a phase of acute denial, but that in this case, guilt feelings could create psychiatric problems later if the respirator were turned off at the father's initiative. He pointed out, however, that there are reported cases of guilt on the part of parents who take an infant diagnosed trisomy-18 from the hospital only to have it die under their care.

The psychiatric social worker reported that contrary to the psychiatrist's characterization of the father, she felt that, in general, the family would be put under extreme stress if the infant were brought home.

At this point in the conference a nurse who had been responsible for the care of the infant while it was in the nursery expressed her outrage. She said that the infant could not be allowed to die by the hand of man but must be given every chance to live. In fact, the nurse said, if no one else would care for the infant, she would do everything to try to adopt her and care for her herself. The Code of Ethics for nurses states: "The nurse's primary commitment is to the patient's care and safety. She must be alert to take appropriate action regarding any instances of incompetent, unethical or illegal practice by any member of the health care team, or any action on the part of others that is prejudicial to the patient's best interests." The code also specifies: "The nurse's respect for the worth and dignity of the individual human being extends throughout the entire life cycle, from birth to death."

Next in the conference a pediatrics resident called attention to the condition of another infant on the ward for whom she was directly responsible. This infant had a slight respiratory difficulty. The resident said that without the respirator the infant would probably have a fifty-fifty chance of some brain damage. She said that she would feel much better if the patient under her care were on a respirator. There were other respirators in the hospital, but all were being used with patients who had a serious and meaningful need for them.

This situation is fraught with moral problems. One obvious ethical issue that must be dealt with is the allocation of a scarce medical resource—in this case, the respirator. Another crucial issue in this case is who, among all of the persons involved in the case, should make this difficult decision. But for our purposes, this case illustrates a more important point, namely, that moral problems in medical contexts are unavoidable. Conflicts arise and decisions must be made. In these situations, no matter what is decided the decision is a moral one. If a physician learns that a patient has cancer and will die soon, the physician must decide either to tell the patient the truth or to withhold the information. Either way, the decision is a moral one. Thus for medical workers, and for all human beings, moral problems cannot be avoided.

## MODELS OF THE MEDICAL WORKER–PATIENT RELATIONSHIP

The very way that the medical worker envisions the relationship with the patient can itself have important ethical implications. In fact, from a practical point of view this may be more important than any of the more specific issues discussed in this book. How the medical worker conceives his or her proper role in relation to the patient will affect all of the moral decisions made in that context. Robert Veatch has discussed three dominant models of the medical worker–patient relationship.[5] Each of these models establishes an ideal of how the medical worker–patient relationship should be regarded. None of the advocates of these positions claims that the relationship exists as he or she believes it ought to be.

### Engineering Model

In this model medical workers regard themselves strictly as applied scientists. They believe that they must deal only with facts and must divorce themselves from all questions of value. The role of physicians, for example, is to present all of the facts to their patients, let them make their own decisions and carry out those wishes for their patients. Physicians are to make no value judgments about their patients' decisions. Or more accurately, physicians must not let their value judgments affect their actions in medical contexts. On this view, then, a Roman Catholic physician, who in his private life believes that abortion is an act of murder, should have no qualms about performing an abortion for a patient who requests it. This is his role as an applied scientist. A desirable feature of the engineering model is that the medical worker does regard the patient as an autonomous being capable of making decisions. But there are three undesirable features of this model which make it an inappropriate way to conceive the medical worker–patient relationship.

First, it is impossible for medical workers to make no value judgments. Medical workers, and all other people as well, are put in situations where they are forced to make and act on value judgments. In some situations, any decision made is a value judgment (Cases 3 and 4, for example). Second, it is undesirable to force a medical worker to participate in an act understood to be immoral. Not only is this unfair to the medical worker, but nobody should be encouraged to perform actions that are considered morally heinous to him or her. In the example of the Roman Catholic physician, certainly this person should not be encouraged to perform acts believed by him to be murderous. In effect, then, these first two criticisms of the engineering model deny its claim of value neutrality. A number of value judgments, regarding telling the truth, going along with the patient's wishes on abortion, and the like, are embedded in it. The third criticism is that this model presents an unrealistic picture of science. In saying that the medical worker should be nothing but an applied scientist, the myth is perpetuated that scientists qua scientists make no value judgments. This is surely false. Scientists do make value judgments. The very act of deciding that a certain research project is worth pursuing is itself a value judgment. For these reasons, then, the engineering model is an inappropriate way to understand the relationship between the medical worker and the patient.

## Paternalistic Model

Also called the priestly model, this view has the patient coming to the medical worker for treatment, counsel, and comfort. The decision-making is placed entirely in the physician's hands; the patient is expected to follow the orders of the medical worker. The function of the medical worker is *always to do what is best for the patient*. The slogan often associated with this model is "benefit and do no harm to the patient." It would seem absurd to attack this principle, but it is used to justify a considerable amount of paternalistic behavior. The locus of decision-making is taken away from the patient and placed in the hands of the professional. As Veatch says, a chief sign of this model is the "speaking-as-a" syndrome. Often a physician will preface his remarks by saying, "speaking as your doctor." Frequently what follows, though, are value judgments and not merely medical advice. Yet by prefacing the remarks in this way, they are given an aura of expertise, an expertise that the medical worker does not have qua medical worker. An expert on medical matters is in no way necessarily an expert on moral matters. This point, in fact, is the first major criticism of this model of the medical worker–patient relationship. On this view the medical worker pretends to be or is presented as an expert on both medical and moral matters. But being knowledgeable about the former does not make a person an expert with regard to the latter. A second criticism is that this model gives medical workers too much power. The ideal situation, according to this model, is to have the medical worker make all of the important decisions. The patient is expected to submit totally to the authority of the physician. Treating patients as if they were children, however, is surely inappropriate. When decisions such as whether to be sterilized, whether to have surgery, or whether to have a limb amputated must be made, surely the patient should have something to say about the matter. If a patient would rather die than live without his or her legs, it seems inappropriate to amputate these limbs even if the physician (and most other people) thinks that this preference is foolish or irrational.

## Contractual Model

This third model of the relationship between the medical worker and the patient attempts to capture the desirable features of the previous two models. Its principal features can be summarized as follows. (a) On this view there is an implied, tacit, lay contract between the medical worker and the patient. The relationship involves a genuine interaction and sharing by both parties. Each plays a role in the decision-making process. (b) There are obligations and benefits for each party. For example, each party should be honest with the other. The medical worker is obliged to perform as well as possible for the patient. The patient must tell the medical worker all the facts about his or her condition, and must stick to, and follow the plan of treatment they have agreed upon. The benefits to each party are obvious: for the patient, the reward is the return to good health; for the medical worker, there are monetary rewards and the experience of professional satisfaction. (c) The patient is free to make all significant decisions, especially all decisions involving value judgments. The patient must certainly consent before surgery is performed (save possibly in emergency situations), for example. Or if the choice is increasing the risks of dying of cancer or having a leg amputated, surely the patient should decide what is feared more. (d) Though on this model the physician is not permitted to take any major action without the consent of the patient, there is no expectation that the patient will be consulted on all technical details. Mundane decisions can be made by the medical worker. As long as the patient agrees with the general goal and has not forbidden some particular means (for example, a blood transfusion), the medical worker may make the technical decisions necessary to implement that goal. (e) Each party is free to end the contract or sever the relationship. Certainly if the patient is dissatisfied with the services the medical worker renders, the patient is free to go elsewhere. But the medical worker must possess this same freedom. If, for example, a physician has strong moral objections to the treatment or procedure requested by the patient, it is unreasonable to force the person to participate in the act. Problems of ending the relationship because of a moral disagreement can be minimized if each party is honest and open with the other. Thus a patient who has religious objections to blood transfusions should make this known to the physician at the outset. And a physician who refuses to perform an abortion should so inform any female patient of that position.

A patient's values and medical workers' values can and often do conflict. The three models of the medical worker–patient relationship differ in how they resolve such conflicts. The engineering model settles all value conflicts in favor of the patient. The medical worker is expected to put his or her values on the back burner, as it were. Those values have no role to play in the practice of medicine, advocates of this model claim. The paternalistic model settles value conflicts in favor of the medical worker. If the wishes of the patient (other than the desire to get well) are taken seriously, this may interfere with good medical practice. The contractual model requires that both the patient's and the medical worker's values be respected. Concerning all important decisions, unanimity is required. Neither party is asked to compromise. If an agreement cannot be reached, the relationship is ended.

Certainly the engineering model of the medical worker–patient relationship is unrealistic and implausible. And for the most part, there are serious problems with the paternalistic model, as was suggested above. However, there might be some circumstances in which the paternalistic model is appropriate. An emergency situation is an obvious example. In these situations the medical worker must act quickly, and in many cases will be unable to determine what the patient's wishes are (because, for example, the patient is unconscious). Since the patient cannot be consulted, someone must act on the patient's behalf. The same thing might be said about a patient who suffers from severe mental retardation. Under normal circumstances, though, the contractual model seems to be the most desirable. It is surely the ideal way to view the relationship between a specialist and a patient. Because the relationship is limited, the specialist is not in a position to know the patient's values and desires. Here the medical worker is expected to act only with the explicit consent of the patient. Perhaps matters are a bit different, however, when the relationship is with a family doctor; after all, the family doctor is in a position to know the patient's values. Nevertheless the paternalistic model, as it has been explained, is too extreme even for this relationship. When discussing specific issues, such as confidentiality and truth-telling, the clash between the paternalistic and the contractual outlooks will emerge. Thus, though it has been suggested in general and very brief terms that the contractual model is preferable, the implications of each of these latter two models will be examined more thoroughly when discussing particular moral problems.

## CONFIDENTIALITY AND CODES OF MEDICAL ETHICS

The confidentiality of communications between medical workers and patients is acknowledged and emphasized in most codes of medical ethics. Yet, surprisingly, there is radical disagreement among these codes concerning the status of the obligation to keep information about patients confidential. In particular, some of the codes state that this obligation is absolute, one to which there are no legitimate exceptions. Thus the Declaration of Geneva, written in 1948, says, "I will hold in confidence *all* that my patient confides in me."[6] And the International Code of Medical Ethics, devised by the World Medical Association in 1949, reads as follows: "A doctor owes to his patient *absolute* secrecy on *all* which has been confided to him or which he knows because of the confidence entrusted to him."

Some of the other codes of medical ethics, however, allow for exceptions to the confidentiality rule. But among these codes that allow for exceptions, there are differences both in the clarity with which the exceptions are stated and the conditions under which a departure from the rule of confidentiality is said to be justified. Perhaps the best known code of medical ethics is the Hippocratic Oath, and concerning the matter of confidentiality it states, "What I may see or hear in the course of the treatment or even outside of the treatment in regard to the life of men, which on no account one must speak abroad, I will keep to myself holding such things shameful to be spoken about." To say the least, this statement is vague. It suggests, by implication, that some things "may be spoken abroad," but it fails to explain what these things are or what the basis is for determining what they are. On the matter of confidentiality it provides no useful guidance at all. Other codes of ethics, however, are much clearer on this topic. In 1959 the British Medical Association issued a statement which claimed that the rule of professional secrecy may be broken only under two conditions: (i) when statutory sanction would be imposed if the physician fails to disclose the information; or (ii) when breaching confidence will be in the best interests of the patient (even if the patient does not realize this). In 1971, however, the BMA significantly altered clause (ii) of this statement. The amended clause says that if a physician believes that it is in the medical interests of a patient to have confidential information disclosed to a third party, then it is the physician's duty to make every effort to see to it that this information is given to that party; but if the patient refuses to allow this information to be divulged, that refusal must be respected. This change was made after an infamous case in which a physician reported to the parents of a teenager that she was taking birth control pills. The doctor's justification for this action appealed to the second clause of the 1959 statement. He claimed that it was in his patient's interests to disclose this information to her parents. In support of this, he pointed to what he characterized as the physical, psychological, and moral hazards of the pill. Among other things, he professed to be protecting the girl from a sense of guilt that she might experience were she to take the pill without consulting her parents.[7] This action was deemed to be too extreme, too paternalistic (though it was judged to be in accord with the 1959 guidelines), and so the second clause was changed.

In 1957 the American Medical Association Principles of Medical Ethics were issued. These principles say the following concerning the confidentiality of patient communications: "A physician may not reveal the confidences entrusted to him in the course of medical attendance, or the deficiencies he may observe in the character of his patients, unless he is required to do so by law or unless it becomes necessary in

order to protect the welfare of the individual or of the community."
According to the AMA Principles, then, one may break confidence if
(i) it is required by law to do so, (ii) it is in the interest of society, or
(iii) it is in the interest of the patient. The AMA Principles are the most
liberal in regard to allowing exceptions to the confidentiality rule.
Some examples will show the sort of exceptions the AMA Principles are
apparently designed to allow. Concerning clause (i), the law requires a
physician to report anyone treated for shotgun wounds or contagious
diseases, whether the person consents or not. Clause (ii) would presumably be in effect if a physician treated someone known to be a mass
murderer. Clause (iii) might be applicable if a patient had confided to a
doctor that he or she planned to commit suicide.

## CONFIDENTIALITY: THE MORAL ISSUES

Through this brief examination of these codes of medical ethics, considerable disagreement about the status of the rule of confidentiality
has become evident. In order to clarify this dispute, three different
questions will be addressed. Why is confidentiality between the medical
worker and the patient important? What kind of arguments or reasons
can be given to support the claim that there is an absolute obligation to
keep information divulged by the patient confidential? What reasons
can be given to support the claim that there are *legitimate exceptions* to
the rule of confidentiality? Responses to the second and third questions
will be critically assessed. A determination will be made of whether
those codes which take the confidentiality obligation to be an absolute
one are more plausible, or whether those which allow for exceptions are
preferable.

   Why is confidentiality between the medical worker and the patient
important? There are two considerations which make confidentiality of
patient-medical worker communications important. The first appeals to
the patient's right to privacy. There is an expectation or presumption
that these communications are confidential. Thus a patient tells or is
willing to give a doctor or a nurse personal information that is usually
not known to others. In effect, the atmosphere is such that the medical
worker has tacitly promised to keep secret any information divulged.
Since it seems plausible to say that each person has a right to privacy,
there are good moral reasons for taking confidentiality seriously.

   The second reason explains why there is a presumption of confidentiality in the communications between physician and patient. It
seems that confidentiality is essential in order for medical workers to

do their jobs. A physician cannot properly care for a patient unless complete information about the patient has been obtained. Clearly there is much information that a patient would not reveal, because its divulgence would be embarrassing, if the relationship were not confidential. It is worth noting that these same considerations can be cited to defend the confidentiality of the lawyer-client relationship. Attorneys cannot adequately represent their clients without full information. Similar arguments are made by news reporters as a justification for not revealing their sources. If they are forced to reveal their sources, they argue, doing their jobs adequately will become impossible.

These two considerations make it plausible to say that medical workers have a prima facie moral obligation not to divulge information about their patients that was obtained in their capacity as medical workers. But can any reasons be given to support the view that this is an absolute obligation, that medical workers should never breach their patients' confidence? There are at least two arguments that might be given to support the claim that the confidentiality obligation is absolute. The first argument presupposes that medical workers cannot do their jobs properly unless their patients are completely honest. The argument then purports to show that patients will not be completely honest unless there is an absolute obligation on the part of medical workers to keep any information secret. Suppose that the confidentiality obligation is not absolute. Suppose that people recognize that there are legitimate exceptions to the rule of confidentiality. What effect will this have on the patient's willingness to divulge information to the medical worker? How will this affect the likelihood that the patient will be completely honest with the medical worker? It is highly probable that the patient will have much less confidence in the medical worker. The patient will be much more inclined to hide potentially embarrassing information from the physician and the nurse. In some cases it may even lead a potential patient to forego medical treatment. Because of the bad consequences of not doing so, there are reasons for saying that the confidentiality obligation is absolute.

There is a second argument to support this same conclusion. As an initial premise, the argument assumes that there are at most a few cases where it is desirable for a medical worker to breach the confidence of a patient. In most situations the question of breaching confidence does not even arise. Given this, if medical workers were allowed the discretion of breaking confidence whenever they judged it desirable, it is very likely they would make more errors (undesirable decisions) than if they kept the patient's confidence in every case. The reason for this is simple.

Human beings are fallible. Because of this fallibility, it is unlikely that medical workers can correctly identify those few cases where breaching confidence is in fact desirable. To minimize moral errors, medical workers should *always* keep the information a patient reveals confidential.[8]

Yet, in spite of these arguments, our intuitions about the proverbial case of the mass murderer who comes to the doctor for help so that he or she can return to the streets and kill again run in the opposite direction. Surely in this case the physician ought to break confidence and tell the authorities. Are our intuitions wrong, or is there something which will resolve the difficulties to which the above two arguments call attention? The following is a suggestion for allowing exceptions but avoiding the bad consequences just mentioned. If exceptions to the rule of confidentiality are allowed, but those exceptions are clearly defined and well publicized, then such bad consequences as patients losing confidence in the doctor can be averted for the most part. If what counts as a legitimate exception is explicitly identified, then patients can be reasonably sure whether the information they give the medical worker may be divulged. In addition, explicitly identifying exceptions will remove the difficulties of the medical worker trying to determine those exceptions individually. Codes of medical ethics can be helpful here by providing explicit guidance. As a result, many of the potentially bad consequences can be avoided.

But how are legitimate exceptions determined? Certainly utilitarian considerations are important here. If there are certain types of situations in which failing to breach confidence will have disastrous consequences, that will be a plausible candidate for a legitimate exception to the confidentiality rule. There may be other relevant factors too. All of the possibilities will not be discussed, of course. But for the purposes of illustration, consider the three types of exceptions stated in the AMA Principles of Medical Ethics. According to those Principles, it is permissible to divulge information revealed by a patient (a) if one is required by law to do so, or (b) if it will benefit society, or (c) if it will benefit the patient. Beginning with (a), is the fact that the law requires it sufficient grounds to justify a breach of confidence? On the face of it, it might seem clear that the mere fact that the law demands information does not necessarily justify releasing that information. The law is by no means morally infallible, and it may be unjustified in requesting the information that it does. Why, then, is this included as an exception? What reasons can be given to support the claim that a medical practitioner is permitted to break confidence *simply because* doing so is required by law? Two reasons might be given to support such a claim. (i) To break the law is to engage in an act of civil disobedience. This is a very serious matter. Since the medical worker is a citizen of the land, and since no society can survive if its citizens indiscriminately reject the law, the medical worker has an obligation to obey the law.[9] Moreover, it would be very difficult for the AMA (or any other medical organization) to advocate publicly such behavior. (ii) In addition, anyone who openly disobeys the law is forced to make significant sacrifices. In particular, those who engage in acts of civil disobedience are usually punished by fines or incarceration. This is a great sacrifice to ask someone to make. Some contend that people cannot be morally required to make such sacrifices. Thus, a medical worker is permitted to breach confidence if it is required by law.

Are these good reasons? It can be argued that they are unconvincing, that the *mere* fact that the law requires a medical worker to divulge information about a patient does not justify doing so. At best, reason (i) shows that a person ought to be very cautious before breaking the law. Certainly civil disobedience is a serious matter; but revealing information about a patient is also serious. This is a decision a medical worker will have to weigh carefully. And though it may be true that indiscriminate disobedience does threaten the very existence of civilized society, indiscriminate disobedience is not in question here. Reason (ii) seems to rest on a false premise. It is true that some actions involving a great deal of personal sacrifice are said to be above and beyond the call of duty. Surely, though, morality does sometimes require great sacrifices. Parents, for example, are often required to endure great hardships for the sake of their children. And given the nature of the medical profession, it is reasonable to say that physicians and nurses are required to make sacrifices too. It is worth noting how far television and newspaper reporters have been willing to go to protect the confidentiality of their sources. Many have chosen to go to jail rather than violate this principle.

It seems reasonable to say, then, that one must examine particular cases where the law requires a breach of confidence and determine in each case whether such an act is justified. What is the proper province of the law? To answer this question fully, of course, is well beyond the scope of our present concern. Many argue, though, that the law should be concerned only with matters that involve the basic welfare of or a threat of harm to others. If this position is correct, then the only laws that the medical worker ought to obey (regarding a breach of confidence) are those designed to benefit or prevent harm to society. Taking this route eliminates reason (a) as a legitimate exception to the confidentiality obligation. The mere fact that the law requires a breach of professional secrecy is not enough; there must be independent justification of the law. Such a justification might rest on reason (b), or perhaps (c). Someone who adopts this position must then examine each law individually.

To illustrate how the reasoning might proceed, consider several examples. There is a legal requirement to report contagious diseases and gunshot wounds. Are these laws which benefit or prevent harm to society? It seems that they are. That medical workers are required to report any case of venereal disease, hepatitis, or other contagious diseases they treat seems quite justifiable. Much public harm can be prevented if contagious diseases are arrested. This requires some sacrifice on the part of patients—knowledge about their medical condition will be made known to some public officials. But this minimal sacrifice may be required since these individuals pose a threat to other innocent members of society. This presumably is what justifies temporarily limiting people's freedom by quarantining them. The requirement that gunshot wounds be reported can be justified along similar lines. That a person has received a gunshot wound suggests that very dangerous, harmful activities have taken place and may occur again. An investigation may prevent future harm—perhaps even save human lives. An interesting modification of this type of case would be a situation in which a family physician knew that the cause of the wound was a perfectly innocent accident and that no foul play was involved. Should this doctor report this as the law requires? It might be argued that the physician is not required to report this case. By hypothesis, doing so will not lessen the sort of harm which the law was designed to prevent. Whether this is correct is debatable, but those who claim that the physician should report the gunshot wound, even in the case of an innocent accident, make the following two claims. First, there is one type of harm that will be prevented if the physician reports the case—the harm that will come to the doctor if he or she is caught breaking the law. And second, one should note the nature of the discomfort that the accident victim will suffer if the incident is reported. This person will be annoyed because he or she will be required to answer certain questions. But, it is argued, it is not the duty of medical workers to protect patients against such discomforts. The obligations of medical workers are confined to matters directly related to health care. The advocate of patient consequentialism will disagree with this; but the critic will maintain that patient consequentialism is an inadequate theory.

Finally, sometimes the law requires that a person report cases of epilepsy to the Department of Motor Vehicles. The reason for this is obvious enough. If someone had an epileptic seizure while driving, the lives of others would be endangered. An actual case similar to this example occurred in 1965 when a bus driver had a heart attack, plunged his bus into the river, and 30 of his passengers were killed.[10] His physician had known about the bad heart and had urged him to stop driving. However, the physician felt that he should not report this to the bus company because his patient would undoubtedly lose his job. And certainly given the nature of our society, if an epileptic has his or her license revoked, this will be a great sacrifice. This puts the physician or nurse under a great deal of strain. On the one hand, physicians or nurses want to protect the health and lives of many innocent people. On the other hand, many argue that the primary obligation of medical workers is to benefit their patients and certainly doing something that causes their patients to lose their driver's licenses or jobs is not beneficial. Because of this latter consideration, it may seem unfair that medical workers must bear the burden of reporting their own patients. In the case of those who operate vehicles of public transportation, perhaps the ideal solution is that the company has an obligation to require its workers to get physical examinations on an annual basis. If this is done, family physicians will not have to face the prospect of costing their patients their jobs. (Of course, the physician employed by the company will be forced to reveal this damaging information; but this situation will be discussed later.) Until such examinations are required, however, the medical worker must deal with difficult cases of this sort.

There appears to be no corresponding ideal solution regarding the epileptic who drives only as a private citizen. This presents the physician (especially a family physician) with a very difficult decision. This is a type of case, of which there are many, that involves a conflict between the medical worker's duty to society and the medical worker's duty to the patient. There is no easy solution to such conflicts.[11] The view called patient consequentialism resolves such conflicts by requiring the medical worker always to favor the patient. But such a view, it might be argued, is mistaken for two reasons. First, it assumes inappropriately that a medical worker's obligations to the patient extend beyond providing health care. A person whose driver's license is revoked does suffer harm, but it is not the sort of harm that is of concern to the medical worker. Second, patient consequentialism either ignores or denies the fact that medical workers are citizens and thus have obligations to society. It can be argued, then, that a medical worker should report the epileptic's condition to the appropriate officials because the danger of not doing so is too great. It may be, however, that society has an obligation to assume some of the burden that the epileptic must otherwise bear for giving up something as valuable as a driver's license. Perhaps, for example, society should provide epileptics with free public transportation given that their freedom to drive is restricted.[12]

The second exception in the AMA Principles of Medical Ethics requires a breach of confidence if it will benefit (or prevent harm to) society. Certainly in some cases this is a good reason to reveal information. The proverbial case of divulging information about the mass murderer is a paradigmatic example. In a "real life" case of this sort, it was a physician who provided the key clue which led to the capture of Richard Speck, a man who was convicted of murdering eight student nurses in Chicago.[13] The doctor in question had earlier treated Speck in an emergency case (while Speck was incoherent). After the murders, the police released a composite sketch of the suspect and stated that on his arm was the tattoo, "Born to Raise Hell." On the basis of this information, the physician recognized Speck as the suspect the police sought and he so informed them, leading to Speck's capture. The physician surely acted properly. What he did may have prevented much harm. But there are other reasons to justify his action.

It might be argued that the doctor-patient relationship did not even exist between Speck and this physician. Because of the circumstances under which Speck was treated—in an emergency room while he was incoherent—no contractual relationship could have existed between them. Yet, even if the doctor-patient relationship did exist, it can be argued that the breach of confidence was justified. When a citizen engages in criminal activities, such as murder, a forfeiture of some individual rights occurs. So if revealing information about a patient who has committed heinous crimes will lead to his or her capture, the medical worker is surely justified in doing so. Like cases involving a person who has a contagious disease, Speck is a *threat* to innocent people; unlike those cases, though, he is *no innocent threat*. That he is not innocent makes the case for breaching confidence all the stronger.

A more difficult case where a medical worker might prevent harm is that in which a psychiatrist divulges information communicated by a patient. An infamous example of this type of case occurred in Texas in the 1960s. A Dallas psychiatrist let it be known, long after the incident occurred, that Charles Whitman had given expression to a fantasy of ascending a tower and shooting people. In fact, after talking to the psychiatrist, Whitman had done this on the campus of the University of Texas, murdering a number of people and eventually being killed himself. The psychiatrist's act seemed pointless since there was no doubt about who the murderer was and Whitman was already dead. In the psychiatrist's defense, however, it might be argued that he was alerting others to be on the lookout for this sort of case and, perhaps, to consider seriously reporting patients who express such fantasies. Apart from this, though, this kind of case raises two important questions.

Should psychiatrists report to officials when a patient expresses a desire of the sort that Whitman did? The answer to this depends on the facts of psychiatry. Some have argued, based on certain factual assumptions, that there are three reasons for psychiatrists not revealing this information. First, they claim that only a small percentage of those who express such fantasies ever carry them out; and the expression of such fantasies often indicates that the patient is improving. Second, among all of those who do express fantasies of this sort, psychiatrists are unable to predict reliably who will act out those fantasies. Finally, if psychiatrists were to report such conversations, this would deter many from seeking help. If these are indeed facts, then the case for not reporting is a strong one. It is important to note, however, that even if psychiatrists should not report patients who express such fantasies, this does not cast doubt on the exception that breaching confidence is justified when it prevents harm to others. Rather it demonstrates how difficult it is to determine when a certain course of action prevents more harm than it produces. Harm may come to others whether psychiatrists breach their patients' confidence or not. Psychiatrists must determine the lesser of the two evils. If they cannot be trusted by their potential patients, then perhaps far fewer people will seek psychiatric help and even more innocent people will be harmed.

The second question concerns what to do in a situation in which a person like Whitman comes to trial. Should statements that he made to his psychiatrist prior to the act be admissible as evidence in court? Again, it has been argued that there are two reasons for saying that such statements should not be admissible. First, there is a sense in which this would amount to forcing the defendant to testify against himself.[14] Information would be used that the patient divulged willingly, but only because of the belief that the communication was confidential. Second, if such a breach of confidentiality were permissible, this would deter many contemplating such crimes from seeking psychiatric help because of a fear of what might happen later. Since many of these would-be criminals might not commit the crime if they obtained psychiatric help, this is an undesirable result. In summary, because psychotherapy, to be successful, must be based on complete trust, it will be very difficult to justify breaching confidence in such cases.

Turning to (c), the third exception in the AMA Principles, is it permissible to break confidence because it will benefit the patient? Such action, of course, involves paternalistic behavior on the part of the medical worker. Suppose a patient tells a physician that he or she is going to commit suicide. May the physician violate the patient's confidence in this type of case? Certainly it would seem that the physician's act prevents significant harm. However, this is not the only relevant question. It is also important to ask if the patient has a right to commit suicide. If the patient is mentally competent and does have such a right, then the physician may not be justified in breaching confidence even though it would prevent great harm. Some may say that even if the patient does have the right to commit suicide, this is not the only consideration. The patient's family has a right to know since they will be harmed (at least in some sense) by the suicide. If this is correct, then this is a case of conflicting rights and the medical worker must try to determine which is more important. Many will argue that the medical worker's primary obligation is to the patient, thus easily resolving this conflict. The issue, though, is more complicated. Certainly the medical worker has a duty to society as well as to the patient, and these duties can conflict. There may be no general way to resolve this issue; one may have to deal with the questions on a case by case basis. Suffice it to say that this conflict between the interests of the patient and the interests of society presents one of the most difficult moral problems in medical ethics.[15]

Perhaps, though, if the only reason the conflict arises is because the medical worker is considering paternalistic intervention on behalf of the patient, it can be resolved. Because factors other than purely medical ones are involved here, it seems reasonable to say that exactly what is in the patient's best interests is not always clear. Sometimes the patient and medical worker will disagree about what is in the best interests of the former because they have different values. When value judgments are involved, the physician is probably not the best judge of what is in the patient's overall interests. Recall the infamous case that led the British Medical Association to alter its statement on confidentiality. This sort of case shows the dangers involved in allowing medical workers to have too much power or say in what is in a person's best interests. If a person gives to medical workers a blank check to do anything that they judge to be in the patient's best interests, their power will filter quickly beyond the medical realm. It seems reasonable, then, to disallow this third exception. The line taken by the BMA seems more plausible. If a medical worker judges that the patient will benefit if others have certain information about the patient's condition, then the medical worker should try to persuade the patient to allow that information to be conveyed to the appropriate people. But if the patient refuses, those wishes must be honored. If the patient is unconscious or incompetent an exception to this claim must be allowed.

## CONFIDENTIALITY AND CONFLICTING LOYALTIES

Medical workers often face conflicts of loyalties, and this can be well illustrated with the issue of confidentiality. Consider the following case.[16]

David, the oldest of three children, was the son of a well-to-do manufacturer. David's father valued physical prowess and athletic accomplishments, areas in which David showed little interest. When David was 12 or 13 years old, conflicts with his father resulted in almost nightly arguments. It was evident that David's father was concerned about David's mannerisms and considered them to be effeminate.

David's schoolwork deteriorated considerably and he became withdrawn. His father decided to send him to a military school, but he remained there for only six months. By this time, David had told his parents that he was a homosexual, had engaged in, and was engaging in homosexual practices. He came home and completed his high school studies, but did not go to college and continued to live at home.

He was treated for gonorrhea, asthma, and infectious hepatitis. At the age of 21, to gain exemption from the draft, his physician attested to the fact that he was a homosexual.

Five years later, Joan visited her family physician for a premarital serological exam. The physician was the same physician who had treated David. Joan was 24 years old and had been under this physician's care since the age of 14. A close and warm relationship had developed between the physician and Joan's family, and it was normal, then, for the physician to ask about her fiance. When he did, he learned that she was about to marry David. She had known him only briefly, but well enough, she felt, to be certain about her choice. Nothing more was said at the time.

David and Joan were married shortly thereafter and lived together for a period of six months. The marriage was annulled on the basis of nonconsummation. David told Joan that he was homosexually oriented, and she learned as well that not only did they share a physician but also that the physician was aware of David's homosexuality. She subsequently suffered a depression as a result of this experience and was angry that her physician had remained silent about David. She felt that she could have been spared this horrible episode in her life—that it was her physician's duty to inform her. His failure to do so was an act of negligence resulting in deep emotional scars.

This is a curious case of conflicting loyalties, a case where the physician must divulge confidential information about one patient in order to benefit another patient. Is this permissible? May the physician reveal what he knows about David in order to benefit his other patient, Joan? In the legal profession, of course, it is stressed that attorneys must go to great lengths to avoid such conflicts of interests. But this sort of conflict cannot be anticipated by the medical worker. The crucial issue concerns what the physician owes to Joan. If the appropriate model of the relationship between the physician and the patient is the contractual one, then this may provide a clue as to what the physician owes Joan. Certainly, if the doctor in question were a specialist, then the doctor's duties would be limited and narrowly defined. It is very unlikely that such a specialist would have a duty to look after Joan's emotional well-being, which is what is at stake here. But in this case the physician is Joan's family doctor, and surely this person's duties are much broader in scope. Are the duties of the family doctor such that he or she is concerned only with the physical health of the patient, or must this person be concerned with the "overall" health of the patient, including the patient's emotional well-being? Given the close relationship between the family doctor and the patient and given the knowledge that the former has about the latter, in normal, nonconflict situations it seems appropriate for the general practitioner to look out for the overall health of the  patient. Surely, though, the primary concern of the family doctor is the physical health of the patient. And in situations of conflicting loyalties, such as this one, it seems reasonable to say that the physician must act only on that primary concern. The fallibility of a general practitioner's judgments in the area of mental health reinforces this view. Thus it would be inappropriate for the family doctor to violate the confidence of one patient in order to protect the emotional health of another patient. Imagine a slight variation in this case, though. Suppose that the physician in question were a psychiatrist, one whose area of expertise is mental health. What would the psychiatrist's obligations be in this situation? This is an important and difficult question that will not be pursued here.

One other case of conflicting loyalties will be discussed briefly. This is the situation of a physician who is employed by a company. This doctor's duties may include giving physical examinations to prospective employees, giving current employees annual examinations, treating emergency cases, and the like. The physician usually discloses information about the patient to his or her employer. That, after all, is why the company hires the doctor. It is possible, though, that the company has hired the physician simply to look after the interests of the employees. In such a case, it will have to be made clear that the interests of the patient will always come first. But when the physician does routinely report his or her findings to the company, this can be detrimental to the interests of the patient. In some cases, for example, a prospective employee may not be hired because of a physical condition. Is such a breach of confidence justified? Or should physicians refuse to work for companies? Some may claim that one should never become a company doctor. To do so, it might be argued, is to violate that clause of the Hippocratic Oath which counsels doctors to keep patients from harm. However, if the nature of the physician-patient relationship in these cases is understood, it can be argued that disclosure of information about the patient is not inappropriate. Here there is no expectation of confidentiality. The relationship is a limited one. The terms of the implied contract between the patient and the company physician are clear and are very different from those with the patient's family physician. In these situations, the patient may even regard this relationship with the company doctor as an adversary one: the physician is looking for factors that will prevent the patient from getting or keeping the job. The atmosphere is such that not only can the patient not expect the communications to remain confidential, but the physician can only expect minimal cooperation from the patient. Certainly the patient cannot be expected to volunteer information which may be used against him or her. Such a relationship will not be a very satisfactory one; for the medical worker the experience may be professionally unrewarding. But given the need for company physicians, it seems that it is permissible for a physician to accept such a role.

There are, however, limits on what the physician owes to the company. Suppose, for example, that a doctor discovers that a company employee has contracted cancer because of working conditions—perhaps the employee is constantly exposed to dangerous chemicals. It may cause embarrassment or bad publicity for the company if this is known. Nevertheless that does not justify withholding such information from the patient. The medical worker may even have an obligation to make this information available to the public. Certainly, though, the patient has a right to such pertinent information about his or her condition. A medical worker involved in what has come to be called "sports medicine" is in a position in which this same type of conflict might arise. Professional football teams, for example, employ physicians. Suppose that the team's star halfback seriously sprains his ankle the week of the team's most important game. The owner may urge the physician to administer cortisone and a local anesthetic so that the halfback can play without pain. However, since such an action would clearly increase the chances that the player might be injured even more seriously, the physician should reject the request.

## TRUTH TELLING

Most people believe there is a prima facie obligation to tell the truth. Lying or intentionally deceiving another is usually thought to be wrong. In spite of this widespread belief, most codes of medical ethics make no reference to the medical workers' duty to be truthful to their patients. One notable exception to this claim is the Patient's Bill of Rights. The second clause of that document is this.[17]

> The patient has the right to obtain from his physician complete current information concerning his diagnosis, treatment, and prognosis in terms the patient can be reasonably expected to understand. When it is not medically advisable to give such information to the patient, the information should be made available to an appropriate person in his behalf.

Here the patient's right to have complete information about his condition is affirmed. However, there is allowance for an exception. If it is judged that it would be medically inadvisable to give the patient this information, then all that is required is that the information be conveyed to some close associate of the patient—presumably a spouse, a parent, a child, or a sibling. Nothing is said about when it might be medically inadvisable to disclose complete information to the patient. Apparently that judgment is to be made by the physician on a case by case basis.

Unless the results of some recent surveys are totally inaccurate, patients and medical workers sharply disagree about whether a patient diagnosed to have cancer should be told the truth. In one study, 88 percent of the physicians responding reported that they follow the usual policy of not telling patients that they have cancer.[18] Patients, however, responded quite differently when asked if they would want to be told that they had cancer. Of a group of known cancer patients, 89 percent said that they would want to be told. From a group of patients without known cancer (and who had no reason to believe they had cancer), 82 percent reported that they would want to be told the truth. And from a group of patients being examined at a cancer detection center, an astounding 98 percent said that they would want to know if their condition were diagnosed to be cancer.[19] Why do physicians and patients differ so radically on this issue? No doubt this conflict of values must be explained in terms of a more basic disagreement. An examination of the different arguments on the issue of truth telling in medical contexts might help us to understand this conflict better.

### Deontological Argument for Always Telling the Truth

Some deontologists claim that there is a duty to tell the truth, period. Telling a lie is not bad because it produces harm; it is simply bad in itself. And, it is claimed, withholding the truth can be as wrong as directly lying. Thus there is an absolute obligation to tell the truth. This position is most often associated with the eighteenth century German philosopher, Immanuel Kant. In one well-known passage, Kant argues:[20]

> The duty of being truthful . . . is unconditional. . . . Although in telling a certain lie I do not actually do anyone a wrong, I formally but not materially violate the principle of right. . . . To be truthful (honest) in all declarations, therefore, is a sacred and absolutely commanding decree of reason, limited by no expediency.

Kant, it seems, allows for no exceptions to the truth telling rule. There are numerous criticisms of this argument, the most common objection being that this position is much too superficial. Physicians manifest this skeptical attitude when they describe the principle as "truth for truth's sake." This criticism, however, requires a more precise statement.

Any plausible deontological system will have a number of moral rules, including the obligation to tell the truth. Surely another of those rules will express an obligation not to cause harm or suffering. What happens, though, if these two rules conflict, as they surely do in many cases, especially in medical contexts? If telling the truth will cause the patient to suffer, how can both rules be satisfied? The deontological argument requires that a person tell the truth, no matter what rule it conflicts with. But such a position seems quite naive and implausible, the critics charge. Surely if a person causes great suffering by telling the truth, then it is not obvious that that person is doing the right thing. The deontologist's argument is too simple-minded because it places on truth telling a value much higher than would ordinarily be assigned to it.

## Consequentialist Case for Withholding the Truth

Perhaps the most common argument to justify withholding the truth from the patient—an argument widely accepted among medical professionals—is the consequentialist case for withholding the truth. The argument appeals to the best interests of the patient, and may be sketched as follows.

1. A medical worker ought not to do anything that will, on balance, harm the patient.
2. In some cases telling the patient the truth about his or her condition will harm that patient.
3. So in those cases the medical worker ought not to tell the patient the truth about his or her condition.

Premise (1) of this argument states the principle of patient consequentialism. It directs the medical worker to do what is best for the patient. Premise (2) makes a factual claim—in some situations the patient will be better off if he or she does not know the truth. What does the advocate of this argument have in mind here? The typical case supposedly covered by premise (2) occurs when the patient is believed to be terminally ill. Why will telling this patient the truth about his or her condition be wrong? To do so might cause a variety of bad consequences: the patient may experience acute anxiety; the patient may lose all hope; the patient may die sooner than expected because of the loss of "the will to live"; the patient may commit suicide upon hearing the bad news; and if the diagnosis of terminally ill is a mistaken one, the patient will have worried and suffered needlessly. Note that all of the bad consequences that might ensue if the patient is told the truth are harmful to the patient. According to patient consequentialism, those are the only consequences that are relevant. Note also that this argument advocates withholding the truth only in those situations in which doing so prevents harm to the patient.

### Consequentialist Case for Always Telling the Truth

It might be thought that anyone who reasons in a consequentialist manner will always say that there are some cases in which there is an obligation to withhold the truth. This is not the case, however. The consequentialist case for always telling the patient the truth has the same form as the previous argument, and differs only in the content of the second premise. The argument is this.

1. A medical worker ought not to do anything which will, on balance, harm the patient.
2. Withholding the truth from a patient will always lead to some harm.
3. So the medical worker ought not to withhold the truth from the patient.

Premise (1) of this argument is the same as before. Premise (2), in contrast with the previous argument, asserts that bad consequences will always ensue if the medical worker withholds the truth from the patient.

The defender of this argument will consider and usually distinguish between the short-range and long-range bad consequences that will follow from withholding the truth. Included among the former are these consequences. (i) In some cases the patient will experience anxiety or general malaise because of not knowing the nature of the problem. This, of course, will occur only when the terminal patient is not told the direct lie, "You are just fine," but rather is told, "We do not know," or "We must do further tests." (ii) Suppose the patient has a terminal illness which is such that if it goes untreated the patient will die very soon, but which if it is treated in a certain way, the patient can extend his or her life by months (and can live a relatively happy, productive life during that time). In cases like this, if the patient does not know the true nature of the illness, the patient will be less motivated to take the treatment seriously. So in some cases in order to get the patient to participate faithfully in the treatments, the medical worker must be completely truthful about the illness. (iii) In many cases what will constitute a rational decision for a patient will differ if he or she is terminally ill. Certainly the economic decisions the patient might make will differ radically if that patient knows that death is near. This is especially true if there are dependents.[21] A person in this situation, for example, would probably not be inclined to make speculative, high-risk investments. A person might also prefer, quite reasonably, to forego expensive, death-prolonging treatment and instead preserve economic savings for his or her family. If the patient is deprived of knowledge of his or her condition, the patient will be unable to make responsible economic decisions. (iv) There may be other sorts of decisions of a more personal nature that patients would want to make if they knew the truth about their condition. For example, a person may want to spend the last days with friends, children, or other relatives. Unless the patient is told the truth about his or her condition, the patient will not have this opportunity. Similarly, a practicing Roman Catholic regards it as a duty to prepare for death by receiving the last rites. And one may want to review one's will, make amends with family members, and the like. These decisions, which are quite important to the person, cannot be made unless the patient is apprised of his or her condition. It is worth noting that considerations (i) and (ii) are medical ones, though points (iii) and (iv) are not.

The long-range bad consequence that will result if medical workers withhold the truth from their patients is that the latter will lose faith in the former. An aura of mistrust will be created. Patients will judge, quite reasonably, that even if they have a terminal illness, the physician will not be truthful about this. Thus when they are told that they do not have a serious medical problem, this will offer them little relief. And even if patients are being told the truth—that they do not have a terminal illness—the patients themselves will be unable to judge whether this is one of the many cases in which the physician is lying. Thus if physicians adopt the practice of lying to their patients when the diagnosis is terminal illness, they will be unable to give comfort to patients who have reason to believe that they are terminally ill but in fact are not. One additional consequentialist point should be made. It is important to realize that most physicians are not experts in judging how a patient will respond to the news that he or she has a serious illness. In this area, their judgments are quite fallible. If they try to specify the cases where patients will respond badly when they are told the truth, more than likely they will err. These considerations strongly suggest, then, that the medical worker ought to tell the patient the truth about his or her condition.[22]

How can there be a consequentialist argument for withholding the truth from the patient and a consequentialist argument for telling the patient the truth? Each of these arguments appeals to the same moral principle. How, then, do they arrive at different conclusions? The disagreement between these two arguments can be seen when examining the second premise of each. In effect, advocates of these two arguments disagree about the facts. Or, to put the point more accurately, they disagree about how to weigh the total consequences. Defenders of the first argument claim that when the total consequences are assessed, there are some situations where it is better to withhold the truth. Advocates of the latter argument maintain that when all of the consequences are taken into account, especially long-range consequences, it is always better to tell the truth.

## Contract Argument

Perhaps the strongest argument against withholding information from patients about their conditions is the *contract* argument.[23] This argument is predicated on the assumption that the contractual model is the appropriate way to understand the medical worker–patient relationship. In normal circumstances the implied understanding between the physician and the patient is that the latter will receive from the former any information which is potentially useful or meaningful. In a real sense, that is why a patient consults a medical worker in the first place. It is obvious, of course, that a prognosis of terminal illness is quite useful and meaningful to the patient; note the consequentialist argument for telling the truth. So the physician has an obligation to present any such findings to the patient, an obligation arising because of an implied promise or contractual relation with the patient. An appeal might also be made to the patient's right to self-determination to show that the medical worker has an obligation to be truthful. The patient, as a competent adult, has a right to make all important decisions affecting his or her life. But, clearly, unless the patient has all of the important information about his or her condition, informed decisions cannot be made. As noted earlier, part of the contractual understanding between the medical worker and the patient is that the latter make all of the significant decisions, and this requires that the medical worker be truthful.

Taken together, the consequentialist argument for being truthful with the patient and the contract argument make a very strong case. At the very least, they show that there is a strong prima facie obligation to tell the patient the truth about his or her condition. It is important to realize, though, that these are very different arguments. The consequentialist argument appeals to what will benefit the patient and says nothing about the patient's rights, such as the right to self-determination. This argument is compatible with the paternalistic model of the medical worker–patient relationship. By contrast, the contract argument appeals to the rights of the patient, and is not compatible with the paternalistic model. Each of these arguments is appealing, and the fact that they are based on very different assumptions shows that there are several good reasons for being truthful with the patient.

### Exceptions to the Truth-Telling Rule

It does not follow from this, however, that the obligation to be truthful with the patient is absolute. Exceptions to this general rule might arise. Ironically, one possible exception appeals to the contractual relationship between the medical worker and the patient. The case in question arises when the relationship is very limited or narrow, such as the relationship between a specialist and a patient. The patient typically comes to a specialist for a very specific purpose. It would be inappropriate— perhaps it would even be considered meddling—if the physician delved into areas other than what the patient requested. The terms of their contract limit the areas in which the physician can be involved. Consider the following case.[24]

> Martha Lawrence was tense and nervous when she came to the Human Genetics Unit on December 12, 1971. She had been referred by her own physician because, unexpectedly pregnant at the age of 41, she was considered a risk for the birth of a Mongoloid child. She was eighteen weeks pregnant, which would not leave much time for a potential abortion.
>
> Down's syndrome or Mongoloid babies are twenty times as likely to be born to women over 40 as to women under 25. About 50 percent of all such babies are born to mothers over 35, and 25 percent to mothers over 50.
>
> Mrs. Lawrence's first two pregnancies had been uncomplicated, and her two sons, ages 16 and 13, were both in good health. The genetic counselor, Dr. Brenda Gould, recommended amniocentesis, the withdrawal of a sample of the amniotic fluid surrounding the fetus, drawn from the abdomen with a needle. The fluid contains enough fetal cells for biochemical or chromosomal analysis.
>
> The sample showed that the fetus had no extra twenty-first chromosome and thus was free of translocational Mongolism. But the sex chromosomes, rather than beeing XX for female or XY for male, showed the abnormal XYY composition. Some research suggests that XYY males might be "supermales," inclined to violent acts, including sexual offenses, while other recent studies do not

confirm this finding. Considering the inconclusive nature of such research, the possible danger to society and the Lawrence family, and the impact of the information on the way the Lawrences might treat the child, Dr. Gould faced a dilemma: what to tell Mrs. Lawrence.

Even if Dr. Gould were to decide this case solely by consequentialist reasoning, the outcome is questionable. On the one hand, if Dr. Gould does reveal this information to Mrs. Lawrence, there is the worry that the child will be treated differently, and because of this different treatment violent, antisocial behavior will result. When taking into account the inconclusive nature of the studies regarding this genetic abnormality, this worry grows more bothersome. On the other hand, if Dr. Gould does not tell her, she will be unprepared and may experience difficulty in handling the boy (should he turn out to be a "supermale").

But consequenialist reasoning may not be appropriate for this situation anyway. In this case an appeal to the contractual relationship to justify the physician's withholding such information from the patient might be made. The patient came to the specialist for a very specific piece of information; she wanted to know if she was carrying a Mongoloid child. Her purpose, presumably, set strict limits on the relationship. Still, this does not seem right. Perhaps Mrs. Lawrence would like to have the additional information. She simply is not in a position to know what questions to ask.

In response to this, two things can be said. First, she could have requested, at the outset of the visit, that she be informed of any significant finding that Dr. Gould might make. Such a request would broaden considerably the nature of their relationship. Second, whenever a patient visits a specialist, it is routine medical practice (well-known to the patient) to send a complete report to the patient's family physician. Since the relationship with a family doctor is much different from that with a specialist, the general practitioner is certainly permitted (and probably required) to convey this additional information to the patient. Still, since the patient is going to receive the information anyway, what difference does it make whether the specialist or the family doctor conveys it? But it does make a difference. To allow a specialist to meddle in areas outside the purpose of the visit is to invite trouble and the return of a dangerous sort of paternalism. Thus the specialist may withhold information, though that information should be relayed to the patient by the family doctor. The contract case for withholding the truth, then, is not really an exception to the truth telling rule. Instead, it tells us the manner in which patients should receive information. This case involving Mrs. Lawrence is made more difficult, however, because of the inconclusive nature of the studies involving this chromosomal abnormality.

Are there any other possible exceptions to the rule that a medical worker ought to be truthful with patients.[25] Of those that have been suggested, several exceptions will be examined to determine their plausibility. Some argue that if the family requests it, the medical worker may withhold the truth from a patient. Typically arising when it is discovered that a family member has a terminal illness and will die very soon, the family asks that the prognosis be withheld so that the patient can "die in peace." Should the wishes of the family members be honored? It may be questioned why the family should be given this information before it is given to the patient. Isn't this an unjustifiable breach of confidence (unless, of course, the patient agreed to it in advance)? And what reason is there to agree to the family's request? Presumably the argument involves an appeal to the best interests of the patient. The family members know the patient best, and if they judge that there would be harm done by telling the patient the truth about his or her condition, they are probably correct. On the other hand, no matter how the actions in question are disguised, they are very paternalistic in nature. If the patient has a right to self-determination, as competent adults do, that right cannot be waived on behalf of the patient even by a spouse, children, or other relatives. In addition, the argument for allowing this as an exception assumes, naively, that the motivations of the family members will always be pure and altruistic, and this may not be so. Though this is a difficult case, these considerations show that this is not a legitimate exception to the truth telling rule. It could only count as a legitimate exception if the patient explicitly gave family members the right to make all decisions concerning him or her.

Another possible exception to the rule that medical workers ought to be truthful with patients is when the patient requests that the truth be withheld. Suppose that the patient says, "Doctor, if it is cancer I do not want to know." Does such a request justify withholding information? To illustrate the difficulties involved here, consider the following case.[26] Suppose that a thirty-eight year old man, Jones, has a wife and three dependent children. Jones owns a real estate firm and frequently speculates in housing development projects. For the first time in many years, he goes to his family physician for a check up. As the examination begins, Jones tells the doctor that he is sure he is in good health, but he adds that if the physician really does find something, he does not want to be troubled by being told. After many tests, the physician determines that Jones has a serious illness, normally fatal in six to eight months. Very little treatment is possible for this disease. Given the patient's plea, what should the physician do? The physician realizes that in avoiding the burden of a fatal diagnosis, the patient is jeopardizing the welfare of his family. And if he is currently considering investments of a highly speculative nature, he could seriously harm his family. It seems reasonable to say that Jones is wrong to make such a request. When the welfare of others is at stake, there is a moral obligation to face all medical facts. Thus Jones is violating a duty to his family.

But what is the *physician's* obligation, given Jones' request? There are at least two different (and incompatible) lines of argument that might be pursued here. The first line of argument appeals to the contractual nature of the physician–patient relationship. According to this view, a physician should initially refuse to enter into such a relationship. It should be clear to any medical worker that a patient like Jones, who makes such a request, is putting the welfare of his family in danger. The medical worker should not participate in an immoral act. By telling the patient that he or she will not honor such a request, the physician gives the patient the option of seeking out someone else's services. The second line of argument, on the other hand, counsels the physician to comply with the patient's wishes. According to this view the doctor faces the classic conflict between an obligation to the patient and an obligation to prevent harm to others. As a version of patient consequentialism, this second line of argument says that the physician's chief obligation is to the patient. So whether the fact that the patient has requested that the truth be withheld justifies the medical worker in doing so depends on which of these two lines of argument is more plausible.

It is worth noting that if the patient has no dependents—suppose that Jones was a bachelor—then the case is a different one. There will be no harm to others and, it seems, no moral objection if the physician withholds the truth from Jones at his own request. The only grounds possible for claiming that Jones' request is wrong, even in this situation, would be if one held that the right to self-determination is an inalienable right, a right that cannot be waived by its possessor. Unless that right is this strong, however, it would seem that there are no grounds for objecting to Jones' request or for honoring that request. Jones may be doing something wrong, however. By putting oneself entirely in the hands of another, one is asking that other person to make difficult decisions. A person who asks another to make decisions about his or her basic health care may be abdicating personal responsibility.

Another possible exception to the truth telling rule is this. Suppose that withholding the truth will not harm the patient and will benefit medical science. Two examples come to mind here. The first is that of "ghost surgery," the practice of someone other than the doctor of record performing surgery without the patient's knowledge. The surrogate surgeon may be a resident or an intern, and this normally occurs when the operation is simple. The second is the practice of medical students giving patients routine examinations but failing to identify themselves as medical students. The impression is created that they are already doctors. In each of these types of cases, it is argued, the following conditions apply: (1) there is no risk of harm to the patient; (2) there will be benefits to medical science; and (3) these benefits could not be achieved if the patient were told the truth.

It is claimed that (1) is true because in each case the service performed is routine, and performable by any resident, intern, or advanced medical student. It is claimed that (2) is true because this provides medical students and residents with much needed training. Without this opportunity, obtaining proper preparation for their profession would be nearly impossible. And the truth of (3) is defended on the grounds that many patients would refuse treatment if they were told the truth because they believe, irrationally, that they will not be treated adequately by an intern or advanced medical student. The major objection to this argument is that the practices in question violate the patient's right to self-determination even if the patient is not harmed. Information is being withheld in order to get a patient to do something that that patient might otherwise not have agreed to. This is a case of manipulation. Since a patient has a right to make decisions about matters that directly affect his or her life, these practices are wrong, even if no harm is done to the patient. This is a powerful objection to the argument that patients may be deceived in order to benefit medical science. It shows that it is not a legitimate exception to the truth telling rule. Still, it is desirable that the benefits in question be achieved. This would best be accomplished if steps were taken to educate the general public, making it clear that certain procedures can be performed by residents and medical students, and that in any case the work of these people is carefully monitored by experienced physicians. If such a program is successful, the benefits can be achieved without withholding information from the patient.

Let us consider another type of case that some have thought is a legitimate exception to the truth-telling rule—the situation in which disastrous consequences will ensue if the medical worker is truthful with the patient. Any plausible moral theory must take into account the consequences of an act; even most nonutilitarians agree that this is a morally relevant consideration. It is quite reasonable, then, to say that in extreme cases a medical worker ought to withhold the truth in order to prevent harm. Consider the following sort of case.[27] A terrible automobile accident occurred. Among those involved were a woman and her young daughter. The daughter was killed instantaneously and the woman was seriously injured. The woman needed surgery and was rushed to the hospital. At the hospital she regained consciousness just before she was to be taken to the operating room. She pleaded with the nurses around her to tell her about the condition of her daughter. They judged that if she were told the truth it would have adverse effects on her—she might go into shock, her chances of living through the surgery would be diminished, and she might lose "the will to live." Based on this belief, the nurses did not tell her the truth. Instead, they told her that the daughter was taken to another hospital and that they did not know about her condition. They made their decision because they believed that disastrous consequences would ensue if the patient were told the truth.

There is little doubt that in cases like this a medical worker is inclined to withhold the truth. In considering this matter, it is worth noting that even if the case in question is a legitimate exception to the truth telling rule, it is not a case in which the medical worker is permitted to withhold the truth from the patient about his or her own condition. In this case, the information withheld is about another patient. It should also be noted that if it is permissible to withhold the truth in order to prevent disastrous consequences, the proverbial problem of "drawing the line" must be faced. How disastrous do the consequences have to be before the medical worker may withhold the truth from the patient? And how do probabilities figure in here? These are important practical problems that will be left unsolved for now.

## SUMMARY

The nature of the obligation to keep information divulged by a patient confidential and the strength of the obligation to be truthful with a patient were the two major issues addressed in this chapter. There is disagreement about whether the confidentiality obligation is absolute. Those who maintain that this obligation is absolute cite two considerations in support of that claim: the bad consequences that will ensue if patients believe that there are exceptions to the confidentiality rule and the fact that medical workers will be unable to identify correctly the few exceptions that there might be. Many, though, argue that there are legitimate exceptions to the obligation to keep information learned about patients as a medical worker confidential. Three possible exceptions to the rule were examined: that the law requires the medical worker to breach confidence; that doing so will benefit or prevent harm to society; and that the patient will benefit in certain situations if confidential information is revealed. It was argued that the first and third of these are not legitimate exceptions. The second of the three seems the most defensible, though in practice it is very difficult to determine when breaching confidence prevents more harm than it brings about.

There is a similar debate concerning the obligation to be truthful with patients. Two arguments, the consequentialist argument and the contract argument, present a strong case for always telling the patient the truth about his or her condition. Since these two arguments are predicated on different models of the medical worker–patient relationship—the former, on the paternalistic model; the latter, on the contractual model—it makes the case for complete honesty even stronger. Nevertheless it has been suggested that there are exceptions to this rule too. One possibility concerns the situation in which a specialist discovers something about a patient's condition, but the information discovered is not what the patient sought. As seen, however, this does not support keeping the information from the patient; rather it cautions us about how the information should be divulged. Other candidates for exceptions to the rule include (i) that the family requests that the truth be withheld, (ii) that the patient requests that the truth be withheld, (iii) that withholding the truth will not harm the patient and will benefit medical science, and (iv) that withholding the truth will prevent disastrous consequences. The pros and cons of allowing each of these as an exception were discussed at length.

## CASE STUDY–1

Prosenjit Poddar and Tatiana Tarasoff, students at the University of California at Berkeley, had been dating. Poddar became very depressed when Tarasoff told him that she did not regard the relationship as a serious one. He went to Dr. Lawrence Moore, a psychologist at the university, for therapy. In August of 1969 Poddar told Moore that he was going to kill his former girl friend when she returned to the country—Tarasoff was visiting in Brazil that summer. Though Poddar did not name her, Moore could easily have determined her identity. Moore decided that Poddar should be committed to a mental hospital for observation. He sent a letter to the campus police asking for their help in securing Poddar's confinement. Poddar was taken into custody, but the police decided that he was rational and released him because he promised to stay away from Miss Tarasoff. When the police informed Dr. Moore about his release, Moore's superior, Dr. Harvey Powelson, ordered that no further action be taken. On October 27, 1969, Poddar killed Tarasoff.

Miss Tarasoff's parents brought suit against the university regents, the campus police, and Drs. Moore and Powelson. They argued that the doctors and the police had an obligation to warn them about Poddar's threats against their daughter. The Supreme Court of California, in a split decision issued in 1976, ruled that a doctor treating a mentally ill patient does have a duty to warn third parties if the patient indicates that he intends to do harm to them. The author of the majority opinion, Justice Mathew Tobriner, argued that the public safety outweighs the importance of confidentiality. Justice William Clark, in a dissenting opinion, argued that confidentiality between the psychiatrist and the patient must always be respected.[28]

## Discussion Questions

1. Looking at this case from the moral rather than the legal perspective, who is right? Does the majority opinion represent the morally preferable position or is the minority opinion more defensible? Why?
2. Dr. Moore could have taken any one of at least three courses of action. He could have kept what Poddar told him to himself, he could have informed only the campus police, or he could have informed the police and the Tarasoffs. Which course of action should he have taken and why?
3. Does the fact that a murder was actually committed in this case make a difference in what the therapist should have done? If there were a case similar to this in which the patient did not perform the

violent act and was cured, would a doctor who kept the information about the threat to himself have acted properly?

4.  What are the similarities and the differences between this case and the one involving Charles Whitman (discussed earlier)?

## CASE STUDY–2

A five-year-old girl has been a patient for three years with renal failure secondary to glomerulonephritis. The girl has been on dialysis, but renal transplantation is being considered. Whether the kidney transplantation will be effective is not known; to attempt it, however, seems better than subjecting the girl to a lifetime of dialysis treatments. The results of tissue typing the patient indicate that she will be difficult to match. Her brother and sister are judged to be too young to serve as donors, and tests show that the mother is not histocompatible. The girl's father is compatible, though. The father then undergoes an arteriogram and it is revealed that he has anatomically favorable circulation for transplantation. The nephrologist informs the father of these results and that his daughter's prognosis is uncertain. After some reflection, the father decides not to donate one of his kidneys to his daughter. He admits that he is afraid to give up one of his kidneys. However, the father does not want his family to know that he has refused to donate. He fears that they will think of him as a coward and will blame him for any of the girl's subsequent medical problems. In effect, if the physician tells the others the truth, he reasons that it will ruin his family life. Therefore he asks the doctor to tell his family that he is not histocompatible. The physician agrees to report to the family that the father should not donate a kidney for medical reasons.[29]

## Discussion Questions

1.  Has the father acted wrongly in refusing to donate his kidney to his daughter? If so, what moral rule has he violated?

2.  A moral problem involves conflicting considerations. What factors make this case a moral problem for the physician?

3.  Did the physician act properly in complying with the father's request? Why?

4.  In this case the physician cannot comply with the father's request by merely withholding information from the family; he must actually deceive them. Does this make a moral difference?

## SUGGESTIONS FOR FURTHER READING

Tom L. Beauchamp and James F. Childress, *Principles of Biomedical Ethics* (New York: Oxford University Press, 1979), pp. 201–225.

Sissela Bok, *Lying: Moral Choices in Public and Private Life* (New York: Pantheon Books, 1978), pp. 220–241.

Howard Brody, *Ethical Decisions in Medicine* (Boston: Little, Brown and Company, 1976), pp. 36–46.

Allen Buchanan, "Medical Paternalism," *Philosophy & Public Affairs*, Vol. 7 (1978), pp. 370–390.

Neil F. Chayet, "Confidentiality and Privileged Communication," in Samuel Gorovitz *et al.* (eds.), *Moral Problems in Medicine*, pp. 85–86.

Joseph Collins, "Should Doctors Tell the Truth?" in Thomas A. Mappes and Jane S. Zembaty (eds.), *Biomedical Ethics* (New York: McGraw-Hill Book Company, 1981), pp. 64–67.

Henry A. Davidson, "Role of Physician and Breach of Confidence," in *Moral Problems in Medicine*, pp. 87–90.

Donald Oken, "What to Tell Cancer Patients," in *Moral Problems in Medicine*, pp. 109–116.

Robert M. Veatch, *Case Studies in Medical Ethics* (Cambridge, Mass.: Harvard University Press, 1977), pp. 116–163.

Robert M. Veatch, *Death, Dying, and the Biological Revolution* (New Haven, Conn.: Yale University Press, 1976), pp. 204–248.

Robert M. Veatch, "Models for Ethical Medicine in a Revolutionary Age," *The Hastings Center Report*, Vol. 2 (1972), pp. 5–7.

William J. Winslade, "Confidentiality," in Warren T. Reich (ed.), *Encyclopedia of Bioethics* (New York: The Free Press, 1978), pp. 194–200.

## NOTES

1.  See Willard Gaylin, "Foreword," in Samuel Gorovitz *et al.* (eds.), *Moral Problems in Medicine* (Englewood Cliffs, New Jersey: Prentice-Hall, 1976), pp. xv–xvi.
2.  These cases are slightly altered versions of ones presented by J.M. Brennan, *The Open-Texture of Moral Concepts* (New York: Barnes & Noble, 1977), pp. 15–17, and used here with the permission of Barnes & Noble Books, Totowa, New Jersey. The use to which I put these cases—to make certain distinctions—is also suggested by Brennan.
3.  The relevant portion of Sartre's essay is presented in *Moral Problems in Medicine*, pp. 51–53.

4. This case is presented in Robert M. Veatch, *Case Studies in Medical Ethics* (Cambridge, Massachusetts: Harvard University Press, 1977), pp. 36–37.
5. See Robert M. Veatch, "Models for Ethical Medicine in a Revolutionary Age," *The Hastings Center Report*, Vol. 2 (1972), pp. 5–7.
6. The various codes of medical ethics referred to here are reprinted in the Appendix.
7. For a detailed discussion of this case, see Veatch, *Case Studies in Medical Ethics*, pp. 131–135.
8. This general form of argument is discussed clearly and assessed critically in Barry Hoffmaster, "The Reliable Criterion Argument," *Social Theory and Practice*, Vol. 5 (1978), pp. 75–93.
9. Such an argument is suggested by Veatch, *Case Studies in Medical Ethics*, pp. 126–127.
10. See Henry A. Davidson, "Role of the Physician and Breach of Confidence," in *Moral Problems in Medicine*, p. 89. See also, Howard Brody, *Ethical Decisions in Medicine* (Boston: Little, Brown and Company, 1976), p. 46. Veatch presents a different case that makes this same point in *Case Studies in Medical Ethics*, pp. 120–121.
11. For an interesting discussion of this sort of conflict, see Veatch, *Case Studies in Medical Ethics*, pp. 59–88.
12. On this point, see Robert Nozick, *Anarchy, State, and Utopia* (New York: Basic Books, 1974), p. 78ff.
13. See Neil L. Chayet, "Confidentiality and Privileged Communications," in *Moral Problems in Medicine*, p. 85.
14. Chayet, "Confidentiality and Privileged Communications," p. 86.
15. See again, Veatch, *Case Studies in Medical Ethics*, pp. 59–88.
16. This case is presented in *The Hastings Center Report*, Vol. 7 (1977), p. 15, and is reprinted with the permission of the Institute of Society, Ethics and the Life Sciences.
17. See the Appendix.
18. See Donald Oken, "What to Tell Cancer Patients," in *Moral Problems in Medicine*, pp. 110–111.
19. See Robert M. Veatch, *Death, Dying, and the Biological Revolution* (New Haven, Conn.: Yale University Press, 1976), pp. 229–231. Veatch's chapter on truth-telling, pp. 204–248, is an excellent one and I have used it as a guide in my presentation.
20. Immanuel Kant, "On the Supposed Right to Tell Lies from Benevolent Motives," in Thomas K. Abbott (trans.), *Kant's Critique of Practical Reason and Other Works on the Theory of Ethics* (London: Longmans, Green, and Co., 1909), pp. 361–365.
21. For a good example of this sort of case, see Veatch, *Case Studies in Medical Ethics*, pp. 154–155. Veatch, in *Death, Dying, and the Biological Revolution*, pp. 211–218, articulates some of the bad consequences that might ensue if the truth is withheld from the patient.
22. The point about the fallibility of the physician's judgment concerning the effects of telling the patient the truth about his medical condition are spelled out clearly in Allen Buchanan, "Medical Paternalism," *Philosophy & Public Affairs*, Vol. 7 (1978), p. 379ff.

23. See Veatch, *Death, Dying, and the Biological Revolution*, pp. 221–222.
24. This case is presented in Veatch, *Case Studies in Medical Ethics*, p. 137. The contract argument for withholding the truth is discussed by Veatch in *Death, Dying, and the Biological Revolution*, pp. 219–221.
25. Some of these candidates for exceptions to the truth-telling rule are discussed by Veatch, *Death, Dying, and the Biological Revolution*, pp. 240–248.
26. A case similar to this is presented in Veatch, *Case Studies in Medical Ethics*, pp. 154–155.
27. This example was related to me by Cynthia Pickles. This was a case that she encountered in her work as a nurse.
28. See Justice Mathew O. Tobriner, "Majority Opinion in *Tarasoff* v. *Regents of the University of California*" and Justice William P. Clark, "Dissenting Opinion in *Tarasoff* v. *Regents of the University of California*" in Thomas A. Mappes and Jane S. Zembaty (eds.), *Biomedical Ethics* (New York: McGraw-Hill, 1981), pp. 119–127. See also, Tom L. Beauchamp and James F. Childress, *Principles of Biomedical Ethics* (New York: Oxford University Press, 1979), pp. 246–250.
29. This case is presented in Melvin D. Levine, Lee Scott, and William J. Curran, "Ethics Rounds in a Children's Medical Center," *Pediatrics*, Vol. 60 (1977), p. 205.

# 3

# Treatment
# Without
# Consent

This chapter will deal with the topic of treating a patient without consent; the subsequent chapter, with the issue of using human subjects in experiments. These topics are related in at least two ways. First, the notion of consent is crucial to each of these issues. In each case the questions of what counts as informed consent, who is capable of giving consent, and whether one person may ever consent on behalf of another must be dealt with. Second, in each case the issue of forced benefits arises. Concerning treatment without consent, the question of forcing a patient to benefit himself or herself arises; when the issue involves experimentation, it is usually a case of forcing the subject to benefit others.

## PATERNALISM

Paternalism involves forcing a person to do something or doing something to the person without consent for that person's own good. It is paternalistic if a person's liberty of action is restricted for his or her own good. Laws requiring a motorcyclist to wear a helmet are paternalistic in this sense, as are laws that forbid swimming at a public beach unless a life guard is on duty. Withholding information from a person for his or her own good is also a case of paternalism. Thus if a physician withholds the truth from a patient because he or she thinks that the patient wll be harmed by knowing the truth, this is paternalistic. And if an individual acts on another person's behalf without that person's knowledge for his or her own good, this can be an instance of paternalism. If a psychiatrist divulges to the family members of a patient that the patient is contemplating suicide and the psychiatrist does it to protect the patient from himself/herself, this is a case of paternalism.

The classic case of paternalism in medical contexts is treating a patient without consent. There are two situations where this might occur: one is when a patient has explicitly refused medical treatment, and the other is when a patient has neither refused nor consented. An example of the first case is a Jehovah's Witness who refuses a blood transfusion because of religious objections to such treatment. Examples of the latter case include a patient who is unconscious (and so is unable to refuse or to consent) and a patient who is not informed about the prospective treatment. In either situation, the medical worker, judging that the treatment will be beneficial, is tempted to treat the patient without explicit consent. To do so is to engage in medical paternalism.

## THE CASE AGAINST PATERNALISM

Before discussing the issue of treatment without consent, let us elucidate the general issue of paternalism. Perhaps the best known opponent of paternalism in philosophical circles is John Stuart Mill. In his classic essay, *On Liberty*, Mill argues at great length against paternalism. In that work Mill defends this general thesis: "The sole end for which people are warranted, individually or collectively, in interfering with the liberty of action of a particular person is self-protection."[1] If another person poses a threat to you, you may interfere with that person's liberty: but you may not interfere to keep the person from harming himself. To defend this thesis, Mill appeals to two other principles. The first is the *liberty principle*: any interference with liberty or restriction of freedom requires justification. Liberty is something to be valued, and the burden of proof is always on an individual who wishes to limit someone else's freedom. Of course, even though there is a presumption against interfering with freedom, to do so is sometimes justified. Mill suggests that such interference is justified on the basis of another principle, the *harm principle*: the only purpose for which power or coercion may be rightfully exercised over any member of a civilized community, against the individual's will, is to prevent that individual from harming other nonconsenting parties. Two versions of the harm principle can be distinguished, and no doubt Mill intended to be committed to both.[2] The *private harm principle* states that one is justified in restricting a person's freedom in order to prevent injury or harm to other specific nonconsenting individuals. Thus, there is justification for preventing a person from killing, stealing, or raping by appealing to the private harm principle. The *public harm principle*, on the other hand, states that there is justification for coercing a person if doing so will prevent the impairment of institutional practices and systems that are in the public interest. Examples of activities that harm public institutions include tax evasion, smuggling, and contempt of court. Although these actions do not injure any specific individual, they do weaken public institutions. Thus such actions may be justifiably restricted by appealing to the public harm principle.

If a person accepts the liberty principle and the claim that the harm principle provides the *only* legitimate grounds for interfering with a person's freedom, then Mill's general thesis has been established. What are the implications of this for paternalism? It follows that forcing a person to do something for his or her own good is prohibited. Persuading a person to pursue a certain course of action by presenting arguments or reasons why doing so would be rational is permissible, but the use of force is not. And Mill makes it clear that his principle applies to groups as well as to individuals. Thus if consenting adults are engaged in activities that are harmful to themselves but not to others, others may not force them to stop such actions. Mill's position, then, is strongly antipaternalistic.

## THE CASE FOR LIMITED PATERNALISM

Some, though, have thought that Mill goes too far. Surely in some cases paternalism is justified. Most people, for example, approve of legislation that forbids selling oneself into slavery. (Oddly enough, Mill too approves of such legislation.) Recently, Gerald Dworkin has argued that in some cases interference with a person's freedom on paternalistic grounds is justified.[3] Dworkin contends that there are a number of cases where paternalistic interference is justified. What he hopes to do is state the principle that captures our judgments about these cases. The principle that Dworkin suggests, which might be called the *paternalistic principle*, is: We are justified in interfering with a person's freedom of action for his or her own good only if doing so will preserve a wider range of freedom for that individual. This principle applies in a straightforward manner to the case of selling oneself into slavery. In forbidding such an action, a person's liberty is being limited. But in doing so, a wider range of freedom for that person is preserved. If the person were permitted to make this one choice, that person would permanently limit all future options. In denying one choice to the person, other choices are left open. That Dworkin's paternalistic principle fits this case so neatly is certainly a point in its favor.

Parental paternalism is another case that Dworkin's principle accounts for. Certainly in many situations parents are justified in restricting the freedom of their children for their own good. By interfering with a child's freedom, a parent can prevent the child from permanently injuring himself or herself. Or in some cases a child would severely limit future options by making an irrational choice, such as not going to school, and parents are justified in interfering in these cases as well. Dworkin's principle fits here, and certainly in the examples mentioned parental interference seems to be uncontroversial.

Another type of paternalism that seems justified is restricting a person's freedom at his or her own request. A person may want to do (or refrain from doing) a certain act, but knows when the time comes to do (or refrain from doing) the act, he or she will be overcome by temptation or some competing desire and refrain from doing (or do) it anyway. Being so aware of such weaknesses, a person may ask another to force him or her to do what is wanted in the long run; that person may ask someone else to prevent him or her from giving in to the temptation, even if at the time of the temptation that person says otherwise. Homer's *Odyssey* elucidates such a case when Odysseus orders his men to tie him to the mast (and refuse any future orders to free him) so that he will not succumb to the temptations of the Sirens. Similarly, a person on a diet may ask another to hide a certain sort of fattening food because that person has an uncontrollable weakness for that food. In cases of this sort to act on the person's request is to preserve a wider range of freedom for that person: it enables that person to achieve long range goals or desires. Since it is generally thought that interference in such cases is justifiable, indirect support for Dworkin's principle is provided. It is also worth noting that another case of paternalism of this sort occurs when patients ask physicians to withhold the truth from them because they cannot handle tragic news.

Dworkin's paternalistic principle also seems to justify interference when a person's decisions may produce irreversible self-harm. Allowing for some paternalistic interference in these cases might be regarded as a kind of insurance policy against an individual's irrationality. Making illegal the use of drugs that are physically or psychologically addictive and destructive of mental or physical capacities exemplifies this type of case. If a person is forbidden to use such drugs, a wider range of freedom in the future is preserved for that person.

Suicide is another case of this sort. To make suicide illegal is to engage in legal paternalism. Might such a restriction be justified by appealing to the paternalistic principle? Dworkin believes so, though the prohibition may not be absolute. Since the decision to commit suicide is usually made under pressure or stress, it is easy to understand why the decision might not be a rational one. But Dworkin argues against going so far as to forbid suicide absolutely: that would restrict individual freedom too much. Rather Dworkin says that the rational individual would opt for an enforced waiting period; that is, Dworkin supports a law that requires a person to declare his or her intention to commit suicide and then wait for a certain period of time before carrying out the act. An absolute prohibition against suicide is too strict because in some extreme circumstances suicide may be the rational choice to make. Providing an enforced waiting period, however, gives a person time to assess the decision and would likely prevent suicides resulting from temporary depression. Yet how could such a law be enforced? What could be done to get would-be suicide victims to declare their intentions in advance? Certainly the law could be written to encourage people to go through this process. For example, the law might state that the survivors of the suicide victim will not be paid insurance or social security benefits unless the person follows the prescribed procedure. And the law might state that such persons may not be buried in the same way or place as those who die natural deaths or who have followed the procedure. In this case, then, the paternalistic principle allows for an irreversible decision, but only if steps are taken to insure that the decision is well-informed and rational.

Some agree with Dworkin that Mill's prohibition against paternalism is too strict. But some also think that Dworkin's paternalistic principle allows for too much interference. There are far too many cases, the critic will claim, where another individual could plausibly claim that interfering with a person's choices will preserve a wider range of freedom for that person. Rather than trying to settle this dispute in the abstract, an examination of the most common case of paternalism in medical contexts, that of treating a person without his or her explicit consent, follows.

## REFUSAL OF TREATMENT: THE LEGAL STATUS

Concerning a person's legal right to refuse medical treatment, two distinctions are important. One is the distinction between treatment administered in normal situations where the patient can consent to or refuse the treatment and treatment in an emergency room where the patient is unable to consent or refuse. The other distinction is that between a competent patient who refuses treatment and an incompetent patient (or the legal guardian of such a person) who refuses medical treatment.

The law is simplest and most straightforward regarding the treatment of a person in an emergency situation. If a person is incapable of manifesting either consent or refusal, the physician is given the privilege of treating that person, and consent is assumed. Physicians are given the liberty to assume that patients will want that form of medical treatment which is best for their health.[4] Thus even if it should turn out that the patient has serious objections to the form of treatment that the doctor administered, no law has been broken (assuming that the form of treatment is standard and the physician is not guilty of negligence).

But what is the legal situation when in normal circumstances a competent patient refuses treatment? May the physician overrule the patient's wishes and treat that person? In cases of this sort there has been a strong tendency on the part of the courts to protect the principle of freedom and self-determination. A mentally competent adult's refusal of medical treatment is not considered unlawful, and in fact must be honored. In 1960 the Kansas Supreme Court ruled on a case in which a blood transfusion had been given to a patient against his will. They argued as follows.[5]

> Anglo-American law starts with the premise of thoroughgoing self-determination. It follows that each man is considered to be master of his own body, and may, if he be of sound mind, expressly prohibit the performance of life-saving surgery, or other medical treatment.

Often this issue arises in cases in which a Jehovah's Witness has refused a blood transfusion even though the physician has warned that it is necessary to save the person's life. Jehovah's Witnesses believe that blood transfusions are forbidden by God's law. They point to certain passages in the *Bible* (Genesis 9: 3–4, Leviticus 17: 10–14, Deuteronomy 12: 33, and Acts 15: 28–29), passages which say that "blood eating" is forbidden, to support their belief.[6] If a person were to assume that there is a God, that God's law forbids blood transfusions, and that the penalty for violating that law is eternal damnation, then that person would have to agree that the position of the Jehovah's Witness is quite rational. Apparently, however, most people do not think that this position is reasonable, and are quite willing to undergo blood transfusions if it is necessary to preserve life. Given this, it might be tempting to force such treatment on a person. To do so, of course, would be a case of interfering on paternalistic grounds. In defense of such a paternalistic practice, an argument might be made that the people in question (the Jehovah's Witnesses) are attaching irrational weights to the competing values in question. Thus medical workers might interfere and force them to be rational for their own good.

Because most people are willing to undergo blood transfusions, they apparently disagree with Jehovah's Witnesses. But many people also agree that religious freedom is as important as the decision by the Kansas Supreme Court suggests. In cases like this it would be wrong to force treatment on people, even when the treatment in question is life-saving. Let us see why this is so. It seems that people are usually reluctant to impose values on others. When moral or religious decisions are to be made, we will go to great lengths to allow individuals to decide for themselves. When possible, evaluative differences are tolerated; in the case in question, no one other than the patient is directly harmed by the patient's decision. It is no exaggeration to say that so much importance is placed on allowing persons to make their own decisions on moral and religious matters that it is regarded as better to decide freely but wrongly than to be forced to do what is right (provided that other innocent people are not harmed). The idea here is stated well by Chaplain Harris of the University of Pennsylvania.[7]

> Spiritual integrity of the patient must be part of the picture, just as physical well-being is part of the picture. In other words, although a patient's religious conviction is one with which you and I may not agree and which may not make sense to us in terms of our own religious outlook, we must consider the fact that it is of central importance to the patient. It is not justifiable to cure a patient physically or give him what is technically the best medical treatment at the expense of his spiritual integrity. In the large sense, the best medical treatment is most simply that which is technically the most sufficient, but that which ministers to the patient's total welfare. The patient's decision not to accept the blood at all costs shows clearly that he is willing to sacrifice his life for the sake of something which he holds to be more precious than life and purpose greater than himself.

The idea expressed here agrees with the opinion of the courts; the rationale providing paternalistic interference on the grounds that the person has attached irrational weights to the values in question is rejected. The right to make one's own religious and moral decisions remains the most fundamental. In 1962 a New York Court put it this way.[8]

> It is the individual who is the subject of a medical decision who has the final say and this must necessarily be so in a system of

government which gives the greatest possible protection to the individual in the furtherance of his own desires.

The courts have consistently ruled, then, that a competent individual may refuse medical treatment on religious grounds or for any other reason. Not only that, but a doctor who performs an operation without the consent of a competent, conscious, adult patient is guilty of battery.

This does not mean, of course, that a person may do anything in the name of religion. In general, it is plausible to say that the state may not interfere with a person's religious *beliefs*. But if a religious *practice* threatens harm to an innocent person, the state may interfere. Thus it is legally permissible for the state to require school attendance, to require that parochial schools satisfy certain minimal standards, and to require that children be immunized against certain diseases; and these requirements are appropriate even if the parents of the children have religious objections to the activity in question. The state also interferes with religious practices in that it forbids polygamy and does not allow the use of dangerous animals in religious ceremonies. Whether these latter two restrictions can be justified by an appeal to the harm principle will be left to the judgment of the reader.

Let us now consider the legal situation when the patient is incompetent. A patient may be incompetent because he or she is a child, is severely mentally retarded, or is unconscious. When a patient is incompetent, someone speaks on that patient's behalf. Thus a spouse, a parent, or a legal guardian may make a decision for an incompetent patient. Suppose that the one speaking on the patient's behalf refuses treatment. Should the refusal of an incompetent patient's legal guardian be honored? Does the legal guardian have the right to reject medical treatment for the incompetent? In discussing this question, two types of cases must be distinguished. The first is when the refused treatment is necessary to save the person's life; the second, when the treatment would be desirable but not necessary to save the person's life. Discussion of this first type of case will be somewhat extensive.

The courts have had to rule on a number of cases in which the parents refused lifesaving therapy.[9] Two very similar cases occurred in 1952, in Illinois and Missouri. In each of these cases an infant was suffering from Rh incompatibility. This is a problem that occurs when the blood from the Rh positive fetus seeps into the Rh negative mother's circulatory system (and it is at least the second such pregnancy). In such a situation Rh antibodies will be produced in the maternal blood, which may cross the placenta into the fetal circulation. Because this can result in the infant's death, it must be given a blood transfusion at birth. In the cases in question, however, the parents were Jehovah's Witnesses and refused to give their consent for the transfusions. The courts, in each of these cases, declared the infant a "neglected dependent" and appointed a legal guardian for him. The appointed guardian then gave consent for the transfusion. It was argued that parents have no right to make martyrs of their children. A similar case occurred in New Jersey in 1962, with a similar ruling. The New Jersey judge argued specifically that the freedom of religion does not give parents the right to risk the lives of their children. The judge appealed to the distinction noted earlier between the freedom to believe and the freedom to act. The right to religious freedom gives people an absolute right to freedom of belief. It does not, however, give the right to engage in any religious practice. And it certainly does not give an individual the right to endanger the lives of nonconsenting adults or children. Thus parents do not have the legal right to refuse lifesaving therapy for their children.

Another case, that of Delores Heston,[10] might be noted here. This case occurred in New Jersey in 1971. Delores Heston was a twenty-two year old Jehovah's Witness, and was involved in a serious automobile accident. Among other things, she had a ruptured spleen. When she entered the hospital she was in shock and soon became incoherent. Thus she was, in the legal sense, temporarily incompetent. Heston's injuries were such that her life could not be saved unless blood were administered to her. The medical team sought the consent of her mother, also a Jehovah's Witness, but she refused. She even signed a release of liability for the hospital. But the hospital applied to a judge of the Superior Court to have a guardian appointed. The court complied with this request, surgery was performed, blood was administered, and Heston's life was saved. We have seen that the law allows a competent adult to refuse medical treatment, even if doing so results in his or her death. The decision in the case of Delores Heston is quite consistent with that policy. Heston was temporarily incompetent and so this was not a case of a competent adult refusing treatment for herself. Rather it was a case of a parent refusing lifesaving treatment for her (incompetent) child. The age of Delores Heston is not the crucial factor. What is relevant is that she was unable to speak for herself and had not previously expressed her wishes. Thus the ruling of the New Jersey court in this case was quite in line with the previous decisions.

Suppose, though, that Heston had previously expressed her wishes. Would that make a difference? A case like this occurred in Illinois in 1964.[11] Bernice Brooks entered an Illinois hospital in 1964 suffering from a peptic ulcer. She had informed her family physician repeatedly over a two-year period that she and her husband were Jehovah's Witnesses and that their religious convictions precluded receiving blood transfusions. She and her husband had even signed documents releasing the physician and the hospital of all civil liability that might ensue because blood was not administered to her. Mrs. Brooks's condition worsened, and she became so weak that she was declared incompetent. Her condition was such that if blood were not administered to her, she would die. However, Mr. Brooks, acting on her behalf, refused to consent to such treatment. Her physician petitioned the court, and a legal guardian was appointed who consented to her being given the blood. After her recovery, however, Mrs. Brooks challenged the court order. She won the suit. It was ruled that since she had unequivocally expressed her wishes while she was competent and since her refusal would harm no one else, her right to religious freedom had been violated. So though Delores Heston and Bernice Brooks were temporarily incompetent adults, the relevant difference in the two cases was that Brooks had expressed her wishes while she was still competent. And, according to the court ruling, the past expression of a person's preferences must be honored.

Are there any exceptions to the law that a guardian may not refuse lifesaving therapy for an incompetent patient? Apparently one exception, when the incompetent is inevitably dying, is admitted. In this sort of case the parent or guardian of a dying child (or legally incompetent) may act on that person's behalf to stop treatment. The treatment will save the incompetent only in the sense that it will temporarily prolong death. This is a situation in which the treatment will be burdensome or useless to the incompetent himself. If no good can come from the treatment, this seems to be a reasonable grounds for refusing it. The courts, too, have gone along with this. The ruling in the case of Karen Quinlan seems to have fit this pattern of reasoning perfectly. Karen's father petitioned the court to be appointed her guardian so that he could authorize discontinuing "extraordinary treatment" designed to sustain her vital signs. Ultimately he was so appointed, and Karen was taken off the respirator. Certainly at the time of the decision it was thought (erroneously?) that the respirator would enable Karen Quinlan to live longer than she would live without it. However, it was believed that she would die soon anyway and would not return to normalcy. Thus her parents were permitted to refuse treatment.

It is interesting to note that the Quinlan case, like that of Delores Heston, occurred in New Jersey (1975). It might be thought that the decisions in the two cases are inconsistent. Since Delores Heston's mother was not permitted to refuse lifesaving therapy for her daughter, why was Mr. Quinlan allowed to do so? In fact, some have thought that these two cases should be treated the same. Judge Robert Muir, of the Superior Court of New Jersey, ruled against Quinlan's petition, and apparently was influenced by the precedent set in the Heston case.[12] Muir's decision was ultimately reversed by the Supreme Court of New Jersey. It would seem that there are relevant differences in the two cases, differences that justify divergent decisions. First, the evidence suggests overwhelmingly that Karen Quinlan cannot return to normalcy. However long she lives, she will be in a comatose state. By contrast, it was clear that Delores Heston could live a normal life after receiving the treatment. Surely this is a significant difference in the two cases. Second, it was thought that Karen Quinlan would not live long even if she continued to receive the treatment in question. In the Heston case, however, doctors had every reason to believe that Delores would live a long time if she received the treatment in question. This also seems to be a relevant contrast between the two cases. And since Heston, unlike Bernice Brooks, had not expressed objections to receiving blood while she was competent, the decision in this case seems justifiable.

It might be concluded, then, that as a general rule a guardian is not permitted to refuse lifesaving therapy for an incompetent. An exception to this rule, though, occurs when the treatment will be practically useless for the incompetent. It may sound odd to say that a form of treatment is both lifesaving and practically useless. However, this apparent oddity disappears when it is realized that some kinds of therapy can keep a permanently comatose person alive, sometimes indefinitely. Surely this is practically useless. Are there any other exceptions to the rule that a parent or guardian may not refuse lifesaving treatment for an incompetent?

Consider the case of a dying child whose life can be saved but only at a cost or burden that seems too great.[13] A case in which just this sort of consideration has arisen is that of a mongoloid child with an intestinal blockage. Clearly intestinal surgery will not be useless to the child. The child will still be mongoloid, but surgery will allow it to live an otherwise normal life. If the parents refuse treatment for the child, undoubtedly it is because of the underlying mongolism. Surely if the child were not mongoloid, the parents would consent to the surgery. Presumably the basis of refusal is that allowing the surgery will result in too great of a burden, either on others (the parents and family members) or on the patient. In the case of mongoloid children, however, it is not plausible to say that saving their lives will be burdensome to the patients themselves. The evidence indicates that mongoloid children do not suffer; they live relatively contented lives. Unless the mongoloid child has some other serious medical problem—for example, a disorder that will require repeated surgery—it seems that the treatment in question will not be too burdensome for the patient. Is it permissible to refuse such treatment because keeping the child alive will be too burdensome to others? Refusal of treatment on these grounds is surely immoral. Refusal of treatment in this type of case might be described as killing by deliberate omission. Certainly we would not approve of other sorts of parental neglect in the case of the mongoloid child, such as failure to feed or clothe the child adequately. These actions are wrong, and so is refusal of lifesaving therapy. Moreover, if this reason is allowed for refusing lifesaving therapy for another, it will open the door to all kinds of possible abuse. This seems to be a situation in which the wedge argument has force, an argument which claims that once exceptions to society's highest values are allowed, further exceptions will follow and these values will ultimately be undermined. These considerations, of course, are moral ones; the legal situation in cases like this, however, is not entirely clear. Robert M. Veatch summarizes his findings when he says this.[14]

> While it is clear that the courts would require lifesaving treatment that would restore or improve the child's health to a relatively normal state, there is virtually no case law giving clear guidance in situations where the treatment would save the life of the child, but leave it with severe mental and physical burdens.

So far our discussion has been limited to the case in which the legal guardian refuses lifesaving therapy for the incompetent. But suppose that the treatment in question is not necessary to save the person's life. Suppose that the treatment in question would be very desirable—it would enhance the quality of life for the person—but is not necessary to save the person's life. Is a parent permitted to refuse such treatment for his or her child? This is a difficult question, both from the moral and legal standpoints. One important issue raised here concerns the nature and extent of parental rights. Clearly there is a limit on the control that parents have over the lives of their children. They may not, for example, refuse lifesaving treatment for them in normal circumstances. By the same token, there is a limit on what the state may do in interfering with the lives of children. Certainly the state may not force the parents to raise the child in a particular religious tradition. The following case raises the issue of a parent's refusing therapy that is desirable but not necessary to save a child's life.[15]

> Jim Powley, a 14-year old, was on a summer vacation with his parents, two older brothers, and a younger sister. They were driving to a cabin they had rented in the country. On the way they were involved in a head-on automobile accident, killing the father and two older brothers. Jim Powley's leg was pinned in the wreckage, breaking the femur in two places and crushing some of the thigh muscle and hip. His mother and sister were cut severly but escaped permanent injury.
>
> Jim spent several months hospitalized while the leg began to heal. For the past month he had been at home, with his mother providing the nursing care. The orthopedist was now recommending corrective surgery.
>
> Mrs. Powley had not recovered from the trauma of losing her husband and two children. She had developed a pattern of praying every morning and evening for Jim's recovery and had visited him daily during the months he was hospitalized. When the orthopedist asked Mrs. Powley for permission to perform the operation, he explained that the risk was minimal. With the operation Jim would have an excellent chance of complete recovery of the function of the leg, perhaps walking with a slight limp. Without it, there was a 90 percent chance he would lose the use of his leg for life. The greatest risk was from the general anesthesia, which, according to the physician, had a risk of about one death in two thousand cases.
>
> After reflection, Mrs. Powley said that even though the risk was small, the thought of endangering his life was horrifying. She refused permission to operate, saying, "God's will be done." Jim said he agreed with his mother.

The legal status of a guardian's refusing nonlifesaving therapy is unclear. Case law does suggest, however, that in certain situations parents do have the right to refuse treatment for their child if it is not necessary to save the child's life.[16] In particular, legal precedents suggest that a parent may refuse nonlifesaving therapy for his or her child if the treatment in question is risky, if it is not obvious that there is a pressing need for the treatment, or if the treatment can be delayed until the child is of legal age to consent for himself or herself. In the case of Jim Powley, though, none of these conditions obtains. The treatment proposed for Jim is clearly desirable and not very risky. Certainly Jim will be able to live a much more satisfying life if the surgery is successfully performed. And in this case the treatment cannot be delayed until Jim becomes an adult. Deciding this case on moral grounds is not easy either. On the one hand, the wedge argument might be invoked to support the claim against interfering with the decision of the parent in this case. If the state is given this much power, then it may tamper in areas that it has no right to interfere with—for example, the beliefs about religion that parents teach their children. On the other hand, it seems tragic to allow the mother's irrational fear of the very small risk involved to affect her son in the way that it will—he will be seriously crippled for life. Would we hesitate to interfere if the operation in question involved no serious risk and was necessary to save the child's sight? Is the fact that Jim agrees with his mother morally important? Would it have the same relevance in the case where Jim would be blind for life if the surgery were not performed? What policy a society should adopt in these cases is difficult to say; the matter will be left unresolved here.

In concluding this survey of the legal status of treatment without consent, let us return to the case of the competent adult. It appears that there are several exceptions to the rule that a competent adult may refuse treatment for any reason. First, judges have sometimes allowed doctors to treat a patient who will not explicitly consent to such treatment on the grounds that the patient really wants to live. Typically this is a case in which a Jehovah's Witness cannot allow himself or herself to consent to a blood transfusion, but it is claimed by the judge that the patient "has made it known" that he or she wants to live. In a case involving a Mrs. J.E. Jones, Judge J. Skelly Wright ruled that blood could be administered to her in spite of the fact that she and her husband refused to consent to such a procedure (because of religious objections). In justifying this decision, one reason that Judge Wright cited was that "Mrs. Jones did not want to die. Her voluntary presence in the hospital as a patient seeking medical help testified to this."[17] In 1965 (in New York) Judge Jacob Markowitz made a similar ruling in the case of Mrs. Willie Mae Powell. Mrs. Powell had refused to consent to a blood transfusion, but apparently made it known that she would not put up resistance if blood were administered to her. Her husband petitioned for a court order for the transfusion. In issuing the order, Judge Markowitz said, "This woman wanted to live. I could not let her die!"[18] In some cases, then, the courts permit treatment without consent if it is judged that the patient really wants to live.

A second exception to the rule concerning treating competent adults without their consent arises when dependents, particularly children, are involved. Returning to the case of Mrs. Jones, one reason given by Judge Wright for forcing treatment upon her was that she had a seven-month old child. The state has a right, he argued, to preserve the life of this woman so that she will not abandon her child. A more complicated case of this sort arose in New Jersey in 1964.[19] In this case a woman in the late stages of pregnancy tried to refuse the administration of blood which was judged necessary by physicians to save her life. The court ruled that the unborn child was dependent on the woman for its life, and so the court gave the order for the transfusion.

There are a number of legal cases which suggest a third exception concerning the refusal of treatment by competent adults. Apparently prisoners are denied the right to refuse medical treatment.[20] Certainly if incarceration is justified at all, then the criminal has forfeited some individual rights. Minimally, the criminal has forfeited the individual right to freedom. But has the prisoner also forfeited the right to refuse treatment? It is not at all clear why the criminal has forfeited this right, especially when the treatment in question is unrelated to the reason for incarceration. In several cases prisoners were denied the right to refuse tranquilizers and other psychoactive drugs. Why prisoners should be denied this right, especially when their grounds for refusal are religious or moral, is far from clear. However, any lengthy discussion of this situation would take us far afield.

## REFUSAL OF TREATMENT: THE MORAL QUESTION

When analyzing the moral issues involved in treating a person without his or her consent, there appears to be an uncontroversial case of justifiable treatment. This is the case when the justification for the treatment is an appeal to the harm principle. That is, if the person is not treated, that person will harm or pose a threat of harm to others. Having compulsory immunization for highly contagious diseases is an example of treatment without consent justified by an appeal to the harm principle. Since the persons who are treated would be a serious threat to others if not immunized, such action is justified.

But suppose that this threat of harm to others is not present. If this condition does not obtain, is it ever justifiable to treat a person without his or her consent? Surely in an emergency situation there is such justification. If the patient is unable to speak (perhaps because of a prevailing condition of unconsciousness) and treatment must be administered immediately in order to save the patient's life, surely a medical worker is justified (and perhaps obligated) to treat the patient. The position of the law that consent may be assumed in cases such as this seems morally appropriate. What about the case of treating an incompetent patient when his or her legal guardian refuses to give consent? It seems justifiable to administer therapy against the wishes of the guardian if doing so is necessary to save the patient's life. There do seem to be legitimate exceptions to this rule, however. If the patient will die soon, or if there is no chance that the patient will regain consciousness, then complying with the refusal seems appropriate. But should the guardian's refusal be honored if the treatment in question would be desirable for the patient but not necessary to save that patient's life? The case of Jim Powley, discussed earlier, raises just this question. What is at issue here is the quality of life the incompetent patient (usually a child) will lead if the refusal is honored. If the treatment in question is serious enough—for example, if it is necessary to save a child's sight or hearing—then there is justification for treating the patient without the consent of the guardian. However, providing arguments to support this position and drawing the line as to what constitutes "serious enough" treatment are matters that will not be pursued here.

Instead the focus here will be on the case of a competent adult in a nonemergency situation; that is, the case of the adult who can speak for himself or herself. Is it ever morally justifiable to treat such a person without his or her consent? Three different kinds of cases that raise the issue of treatment without consent for a competent adult will be described.[21] Surprisingly, concerning the first two of these cases, there is general agreement in the medical and legal communities. There seems to be no such consensus, however, regarding the third kind of case. The approach here will be to examine the reasons given to support judgments about the first two cases and then to see if this forces one to take a particular stand on the third type of case.

The first kind of case—called cases of type (1)— involves a patient who has not consented to but who has not explicitly refused treatment either. So-called therapeutic experiments are examples of this type of case. An experiment is termed therapeutic when a physician uses a relatively new or untested drug or medical procedure, with the primary goal to benefit the patient, not to gain scientific knowledge. Some circumstances are such that the doctor judges that if information about the drug or experimental procedure is revealed to the patient, that patient's health will be adversely affected. Thus disclosure would be contrary to the patient's best interests, the physician believes. In cases like this there is agreement in the medical community that the information may be withheld and that the patient may be treated without his or her explicit consent. This is suggested in part II of the "Declaration of Helsinki" (first drafted in 1964, and revised in 1975), and is stated explicitly in the "American Medical Association Ethical Guidelines for Clinical Investigations" (originally adopted in 1966).[22] Another instance of a case of type (1) arises when an individual is unwilling to consent to a certain kind of treatment but makes it known that he or she will not resist a court order to be treated. As previously noted, the courts have dealt with at least two cases of this sort, each of which involved a patient who had religious objections to blood transfusions. In each of these cases the patient had signed a release of liability. Yet in each case it was said that the patient "made it known" that there would be no active resistance if the court ordered a transfusion. In each of these cases the presiding judge ruled that the transfusion could be administered even though the patient would not explicitly consent. So in both the medical and legal communities it is held that there are cases of type (1) where treatment without consent is justified.

The second kind of case—type (2)—arises when a person objects to a specific form of treatment, usually but not necessarily for religious or moral reasons. The most widely discussed case of this type is, of course, that of the Jehovah's Witness who explicitly refuses a blood transfusion on the ground that God's law forbids it. In these cases the patient makes it known that he or she will actively resist a court order requiring the transfusion. In such circumstances there can be no doubt what the patient's real wishes are. As noted earlier, when the patient is an adult who has been determined to be competent, the courts have consistently ruled that that patient has the right to refuse lifesaving treatment. And, as we previously stated, the person's reasons for refusing need not be religious or moral reasons. If, for example, it is determined that the only way to prevent the spreading of cancer is to amputate a person's leg, the person still has a legal right to refuse such surgery.[23] Such a person may simply prefer to die rather than to live without a leg. The consensus, then, seems to be that a competent adult has the right to refuse a specific kind of treatment even if the grounds for doing so are thought to be foolish.

There is a third kind of case—type (3)—in which the issue of treatment without consent arises. This is a situation in which a patient refuses a specific form of treatment because of a demonstrably false belief. The patient refuses treatment not because of some religious objection and not because of some aversion to that treatment, but rather because the patient is mistaken about the facts of the case. A dramatic example of this sort of case was discussed recently.[24] This involved a woman who was in the hospital because of a fractured hip. While she was hospitalized a Papanicolaou test (a test that analyzes cells from the cervix and vagina for cancer) and biopsy revealed that she had cancer of the cervix. It was judged that the cancer was certainly curable by a hysterectomy, so this surgery was recommended. The patient, however, refused to consent to this treatment. Her reason for refusal was that, in spite of the evidence, she did not believe that she had cancer. She even argued her case: people with cancer feel bad and lose weight, but these conditions did not obtain in her case. Assuming, as was true in this case, that the patient was judged mentally competent, physicians and judges are presented with a difficult problem: Is paternalistic intervention justified in this case? May a specific kind of treatment be forced on patients if their only reason for refusing it is that they have a demonstrably false belief about the facts of the case? Certainly, arguing that the physician has an obligation to try to change the patient's belief is plausible. But if that fails, the difficult question must then be faced. And on this issue, no clear consensus has arisen.[25]

Since there is a consensus about cases of types (1) and (2), perhaps an investigation of the differences between these two types of cases will shed some light on how cases of type (3) should be dealt with. Why is it generally believed (in the medical and legal communities) that treatment without consent is justified in cases of type (1) and not in cases of type (2)? The most obvious and important difference between these cases is that in the second the patient has *explicitly refused* treatment, while in the first he or she has merely *not consented*. The importance of this difference is made manifest by noting how the physician-patient relationship differs in the two cases. In the paradigmatic cases of type (1) the patient has come to the physician for help, has explicitly acknowledged an illness, and has expressed a desire to be cured. The only question concerns the means of curing that patient. Since the patient has consented to the relationship in general, it might be maintained that the patient has tacitly consented to the specific means the physician chooses to employ; or at least he has so consented unless indicating otherwise. Some patients may go so far as to say, "Do whatever you think is best. I do not even want to be consulted." But even if the patient does not go this far, what is common to type (1) cases is that the physician will follow what is understood as the real wishes of the patient. By contrast, the physician-patient relationship is very different in type (2) cases. The patient has come to the doctor with a specific problem, but has stated explicitly that one kind of treatment (for example, a blood transfusion) is unacceptable. The patient enters the relationship only on the condition that the physician will not employ that treatment. One morally relevant difference between cases of type (1) and (2) now becomes clear. When a person is treated without consent in a type (2) case, the infringement on that person's liberty is much more serious than in a type (1) case. In the first case the physician is not really interfering with the patient's liberty since the physician is helping the patient obtain what is wanted. But in the second kind of case, no such claim can be made.

What, then, can be said about type (3) cases, where the patient refuses treatment because of a false belief? In a situation of this sort the patient comes to the physician for some other reason and does not even acknowledge the existence of the illness in question. Given this, there is no way that it can plausibly be said that the patient has consented, tacitly or otherwise, to be treated for *that* illness. To proceed with treatment in the face of explicit refusal would be a serious infringement on the patient's liberty. This suggests that these cases are more like those of type (2) than type (1), and so we might think that consistency requires forbidding treatment without consent in both cases. But it is odd that people are more uncertain about type (3) cases than they are about type (2) cases. To demonstrate further this oddity, it might be noted that our objections to treatment without consent in type (2) situations are antipaternalistic in nature. Yet one of the most stringent opponents of paternalism has approved of interference with a person's liberty of action when that person is acting on a demonstrably false belief. Mill, in Chapter V of *On Liberty*, makes the following claim: "If either a public officer or anyone else saw a person attempting to cross a bridge which had been ascertained to be unsafe, and there were no time to warn him of his danger, they might seize him and turn him back, without any real infringement of his liberty; for liberty consists in doing what one desires, and he does not desire to fall into the river."[26] Similarly, Gerald Dworkin, a defender of some instances of paternalism, suggests that it would be permissible to act against the will of a person who believes that when jumping out the window he or she will float upwards.[27]

It seems plausible to maintain that forcing treatment on a person who refuses because of religious reasons is more serious, from the moral point of view, than forcing treatment on a person who refuses because of a false belief. People are usually more appalled if a physician acts contrary to the patient's expressed wishes in the case of refusal on religious grounds. Surely, then, there must be some relevant difference between type (2) cases and those of type (3). But what is this difference? One striking difference between the two is that in type (2) cases there is an imposition of values on the patient when treatment is administered, but not so in type (3) cases. When medical workers are tempted to force treatment on a person in a situation of type (2), those medical workers believe that the patient attaches incorrect or irrational weight to some personal values. But this is not so when treatment is forced in type (3) cases; in these situations if the person is not coerced he or she will fail to act in accordance with *his or her own desires*. And people are certainly more reluctant to impose their values on others than they are to force them to act in accord with their own actual preferences.[28] It is thought that the liberty to follow one's own moral and religious conscience is particularly (and perhaps uniquely) important. An individual is not autonomous unless free to pursue his or her own values. Socrates went so far to say in the *Crito* (48 a–b) that life is not worth living if a person cannot pursue what he or she takes to be the (morally) good life. It is reasonable to say that people are willing to restrict a person's freedom to follow his or her own conscience only to prevent public harm or to preserve the liberty of others. Because of such an application of the harm principle, religious fanatics are not permitted to kidnap people for the sake of indoctrination and conversion despite the fact that some believe they have a duty to do so.

Minimally, the foregoing remarks suggest that the only cases to which there are legitimate and serious moral objections are those of type (2). These remarks further suggest that despite the fact that initially type (3) cases seem more like those of type (2) than (1), these appearances are deceptive. Type (3) cases are really more like those of type (1). The explanation is that when medical workers act contrary to a patient's expressed wishes when that patient refuses treatment because of a false belief, medical workers are not imposing values on that patient. Let us assume that what the woman with cancer of the cervix really values is her life and health, and she wishes to preserve them. Assuming this, then if she really believed that she had the illness, she would in fact consent to the treatment in question. If medical workers interfere and force treatment on her, they will be forcing her to do what she would really want to do if she believed all of the facts. In some sense then, medical workers will be forcing her to do what she really wants to do. And, it will be recalled, this is one of the considerations that has led some to say that treatment without consent is justified in type (1) cases. Even in the most difficult type (1) case—the case of the Jehovah's Witness who makes it known that he will not resist the transfusion, though he cannot bring himself to consent—the judge's justification for interference involved an appeal to the patient's *real* or *genuine* desires.

Still, there was some hesitation about approving of paternalistic interference in type (3) cases. For this reason, one would be well-advised to examine more thoroughly the reasoning put forward that claims to justify treatment without consent in both cases of type (1) and (3). Recall that in one of the cases in which the patient would not consent to a blood transfusion but made it known that there would be no active opposition, New York Judge Jacob Markowitz argued, "This woman wanted to live. I could not let her die."[29] Similar things can be said about the cases involving a false belief: Mill's man does not want to fall into the river and the person in Dworkin's example does not want to be injured. It would seem, then, that in each of these cases the "interference" is justified because it is not really interference; it is not interference because the person is being forced to do what that person really wants to do. The justification for interference in each of these cases—and hence the justification for treatment without consent in cases of types (1) and (3)—relies on the claim that these are not genuine cases of infringing on a person's liberty. This justification depends on a particular analysis of liberty, one provided by Mill (in the passage from *On Liberty* quoted previously): "Liberty consists in doing what one desires." However, because of the phrase "doing what one desires," this analysis is ambiguous. On the one hand, "what one desires" may refer to the description under which an object is desired. Let us call this the *intended* object of desire. On the other hand, "what one desires" may refer to the real object of a desire, whether or not one knows that that is the object of the desire. Let us call this the *actual* object of desire.[30] The intended and actual objects of desire will be different whenever the agent has false beliefs about what is desired. Thus if a person mistakes a plastic, imitation apple for a real apple and desires to eat it, the *intended* object of the desire is to eat a real apple and the *actual* object of the desire is to eat the plastic apple. Though Mill's analysis of liberty is subject to this ambiguity, what he goes on to say—"he does not desire to fall into the river"—clarifies what he means. "Liberty consists in doing what one desires" means that liberty consists in doing or acquiring the *intended* object of a desire. Thus in cases of false belief, when a person is prevented from seeking the actual object of a desire, that person's liberty is not interfered with.

It is on this analysis of liberty, then, that the justification for treatment without consent in type (3) cases rests. Is this justification adequate? The consequences of accepting such an account of liberty and allowing interference—or apparent interference—on this basis are dangerous. First, allowing others to force us to do something because they believe it will lead to what is really wanted does not insure that the intended object of our desire will be achieved. All humans, no matter who they are, are fallible. In fact, it can be plausibly argued that by and large each person is the best judge of what that person really wants or what is in that person's best interest. Whenever others interfere, they usually interfere wrongly.[31] But, it might be objected, in the cases in question there can be no doubt about what the person really wants; the person has expressed himself or herself clearly on this matter. In these cases, the argument continues, the person has a false belief about what the correct means are to achieving the end. Thus the woman with cancer of the cervix desires to be healthy and to continue living; however, she erroneously believes that a hysterectomy is not a necessary means for achieving that end.

This response leads us to consider a second point against allowing treatment without consent in type (3) cases. Permitting such intervention, even when the only question concerns the means to an end and not the end itself, will open the door to a paternalistic interference usually considered to be wrong. If such a justification is accepted, an argument on the same grounds for the involuntary sterilization of mentally retarded teenagers can be made. After all, what they really want from life is happiness, and whether they realize it or not they cannot be happy if they are saddled with children who themselves might be retarded. Even more dangerously, an argument for forcing the Jehovah's Witness to receive the transfusion can also be made. The end sought is to obey God's law; but the Jehovah's Witness mistakenly believes that refusing transfusions is a necessary means to that end. If the general pattern of reasoning suggested above to justify interference in type (3) cases is accepted, then it would seem that each who agrees that receiving a blood transfusion is not wrong (and presumably this is the vast majority of people) would have to allow interference in these cases. These two examples show that allowing paternalistic intervention in cases of false belief leads to dangerous consequences. It puts us on a slippery slope from which there is no apparent escape.[32]

There is yet a third reason for being wary about a justification for intervention based on the claim that someone is enabling another person to achieve what he or she really desires. In some cases what is really desired is not merely a certain end, but the achievement of that in one's own way. Thus a person may desire a certain job because he or she is the best qualified for it. Such a person would rather not get the position than to have it offered because of that person's race, sex, religious

preference, or relationship to the company president. Liberty here consists of something more than doing or getting what is really desired.
Sometimes *how* an individual achieves an end is just as important as
achieving it. It might be thought that this point can be granted, but
that it has no applicability in medical contexts. After all, people desire
health and are not concerned about how they achieve this end. This,
however, is false. The Jehovah's Witness is a glaring exception to this
claim, and there are surely others as well. There are, then, good reasons
for rejecting this attempt to justify treatment without consent in type
(3) cases.

What has just been argued might suggest that people are never
justified in interfering with a person's behavior when he or she is acting
on a demonstrably false belief, and, it will be argued, this goes too far.
Surely in the examples mentioned by Mill and Dworkin there is justification for preventing the person from acting on the false belief. Since
intervention is permissible in these cases, it must be shown that there is
a morally relevant difference between these cases and situations of type
(3) that arise in medical contexts. Fortunately there is an important difference. In the former cases there is, by hypothesis, no possibility of
altering the person's false belief. In these examples there is no time for
argument or persuasion. In the typical cases of false belief in medical
contexts, however, this is not the case. The example of the woman with
cancer may be taken as a model. In this case the physician has time to
try to change the patient's beliefs. He can present and explain to her
the evidence that shows that she has cancer. Additionally, he might
have another physician talk to her, and he might present the evidence
to her relatives so that they might persuade her. But if all this proves
inefficacious and the patient is mentally competent, then the arguments
stated above show that interference would be unjustified. To see that
this conclusion is reasonable, consider a modified version of Mill's example. Suppose that we prevent a person from crossing the bridge and
explain to him or her why we did so. In spite of our warnings, however,
this person again tries to cross the bridge. Perhaps he or she desperately
wants to get to the other side quickly; or perhaps he or she enjoys high-
risk activities; or perhaps he or she simply does not believe what we tell
him or her. In these cases interferences would be wrong. This suggests
that a morally crucial factor is whether there is time to convince a person that his or her beliefs are false. In addition to this consideration, it
would be very dangerous and a real threat to our freedom to allow
someone who occupies a role as powerful as that of a physician to decide routinely what a person really wants. The bad consequences of
allowing forced treatment in type (3) cases arise because too much

discretion is given to one who occupies such an influential role. If interference because of a false belief is permitted only in those cases where there is no time to change the person's mind and no person occupying a powerful role is given a blank check, then these undesirable consequences can be avoided.

Several remarks about treatment without consent in type (1) cases will conclude this chapter. As already indicated, there are, in effect, at least two distinct forms of jusification offered in these cases; what is common to each is the claim that the practice in these cases is not truly treatment without consent. One justification is that what is being done is in accord with the real wishes of the patient. A defense of this sort involves an appeal to Mill's notion of liberty. The difficulties raised with this defense in type (3) cases are equally applicable here. It is not wise to allow others to say what our genuine wants are. If there is a justification for giving the Jehovah's Witness a blood transfusion when he refuses to consent but makes it known that he will not actively resist, that justification cannot be based on an appeal to the patient's real desires.

The other justification claims that though the patient has not explicitly consented to the specific treatment in question, the patient has indirectly consented. Sometimes this is so because the patient tells the doctor to use whatever treatment the doctor judges to be best; in other cases the appeal is to the notion of tacit consent. When the concept of tacit consent is invoked, it is argued that since the patient has consented to the relationship in general, the patient has therefore consented to accepting the treatment that the physician decides to employ. But surely such reasoning is specious. It is not plausible to say that a patient consents to any means the physician prefers when the former employs the latter for a specific medical problem. At most, the patient might be said to consent to any widely used treatment. However, when the patient directs the doctor to make all of the decisions and do whatever the doctor thinks is best, the matter is entirely different. Here one can say that consent is genuine. Some may object to a person's so unconditionally surrendering autonomy with respect to such an important matter, but it is hard to see on what grounds such objections are based. This situation is certainly not comparable to one in which a person sells himself or herself into slavery. It may even be prudent and rational for some to give the physician such power. If a person knows that he or she often makes bad decisions in times of crises, it seems quite reasonable for that person to take steps to minimize the number of important decisions that must be made during such times. Though the notion of tacit consent remains dubious, nonetheless there are cases where a person has given indirect consent. In these cases a specific form of treatment without explicit consent is justified only because explicit consent has been given at another level.

Treatment without consent in type (2) cases seems unjustified. And since the most natural argument that can be given to support treatment without consent in type (3) cases fails, that is also morally unjustified except in the unusual case where there is no time to present the patient with evidence that the belief is false. How far this conclusion extends remains open, however. Certainly when the treatment in question is as serious as a hysterectomy or the amputation of a limb, then treatment without consent in type (3) cases is impermissible. But suppose that the treatment in question merely involved conducting a test of some sort, such as an X-ray or blood analysis. Whether procedures of this sort may take place against a patient's refusal remains open to question. Finally, treatment without explicit consent is justified in type (1) cases only when it is plausible to say that the patient has indirectly consented. There are surely fewer type (1) cases that are justified than is believed by many in the medical community. Certainly the "American Medical Association Ethical Guidelines for Clinical Investigation" go much too far in allowing the physician to decide whether disclosure would be detrimental to the patient's best interests.[33] Such a license for paternalism is a threat to liberty on any plausible account of that concept.

## SUMMARY

With few exceptions, a competent adult has the legal right to refuse treatment, even if that treatment is necessary to save the patient's life. In an emergency situation, where it is impossible to obtain the patient's consent, the medical worker has the legal right to administer treatment. Indeed, depending on the status of good samaritan laws in his or her state, the medical worker may have a legal duty to provide the treatment. If the patient is not competent, then the issue concerns the right of the legal guardian (usually the parent) to refuse treatment. If the therapy in question is lifesaving, then normally the guardian does not have the legal right to refuse it. There is a clearcut exception to this rule, however. If the lifesaving therapy is judged "practically useless" because it will only extend the person's life for a short period of time or because the person will be permanently comatose, then it may be refused. The law is unclear when the question of refusing lifesaving therapy for a deformed child arises. The law is also somewhat unclear if a guardian refuses treatment that would be very desirable, though it is not necessary to save the incompetent's life.

The moral issue of treatment without consent was also dealt with. Only cases involving a competent adult were considered. It was argued that if a competent adult refuses treatment for religious or moral reasons, it would be wrong to act against his or her wishes. The situation in which a competent adult refuses therapy because of a demonstrably false belief was shown to be more complicated; nevertheless there are strong arguments forbidding treatment in that type of case also. The one type of case where it seems justifiable to treat a competent adult without consent is the case where consent has been given at another level. This occurs when the patient explicitly directs the physician to do whatever he or she deems necessary. When the terms of the relationship are such, the physician has been given the freedom to administer specific treatment without obtaining consent.

## CASE STUDY

Phillip Becker is a 13-year-old boy who has Down's syndrome (Mongolism). A person with Down's syndrome has a chromosomal defect that causes retardation and some physical abnormalities. Phillip has spent all of his 13 years in a home for handicapped children. His teachers say that he is doing very well for someone in his condition; he is able to perform many common chores. All indications are that his life is pleasant. In any case, the evidence suggests that children with Down's syndrome do not "suffer." Phillip also has a heart defect, a situation that is not atypical for children with Down's syndrome. The heart defect could be corrected with surgery. Performing the surgery does involve a 10 percent chance of death. But if surgery is not performed, doctors say that Phillip will die before he is 30. Moreover, the last few years of his life will probably be very painful.

Phillip's parents, who claim to visit him six times a year (though workers at the home insist that the visits are much less frequent), refused to allow the corrective surgery to be performed. The State of California took the case to court in an attempt to force the Beckers to allow the surgery. The Beckers appealed to several grounds to defend their position. First, they argued that the operation is too risky. Second, they claimed that if Phillip lived much beyond the age of 30 he would survive them and there would be no one to assure that he received high quality care. Finally, they asserted that Phillip's life lacks those qualities that would give it human dignity. The testimony of a pediatrician was secured to support this claim. The Beckers won their case in court. And though California appealed the decision, the Supreme Court refused to hear it.[34]

## Discussion Questions

1. In this case the state is contending that the rights of parents do not extend as far as the Beckers believe; the court disagreed. Do you agree with the court's decision?
2. How does the ruling in this case compare with others discussed in this chapter?
3. The Beckers gave three different reasons to justify refusing the surgery for Phillip. Assess each of these reasons. Are some better than others?
4. Unbeknownst to the court, another family had taken a great interest in Phillip Becker. They frequently took him to their home on weekends. They even wanted to adopt Phillip so that he could live with a family. Had the court known this, should it have influenced their decision? Would it have been justifiable to take Phillip from the Beckers and allow the other family to adopt him?

## SUGGESTIONS FOR FURTHER READING

Eric J. Cassell, "Informed Consent in the Therapeutic Relationship: Clinical Aspects," in Warren T. Reich (ed.), *Encyclopedia of Bioethics* (New York: The Free Press, 1978), pp. 767–770.

Gerald Dworkin, "Paternalism," in Richard A. Wasserstrom (ed.), *Morality and the Law*, (Belmont, Calif.: Wadsworth Publishing Company, 1971), pp. 107–126.

Ruth Faden and Alan Faden, "False Belief and the Refusal of Medical Treatment," *Journal of Medical Ethics*, Vol. 3 (1977), pp. 133–136.

Jay Katz, "Informed Consent in the Therapeutic Relationship: Law and Ethics," in Warren T. Reich (ed.), *Encyclopedia of Bioethics* (New York: The Free Press, 1978), pp. 770–778.

John Stuart Mill, *On Liberty* (Indianapolis: Hackett Publishing Company, 1978). Mill's essay was originally published in 1859.

Robert M. Veatch, *Case Studies in Medical Ethics* (Cambridge, Mass.: Harvard University Press, 1977), pp. 303-316.

Robert M. Veatch, *Death, Dying, and the Biological Revolution* (New Haven, Conn.: Yale University Press, 1976), pp. 116-163.

## NOTES

1. John Stuart Mill, *On Liberty* (Indianapolis: Hackett Publishing Company, 1978), p. 9. Mill's essay was first published in 1859.
2. On this point, see Joel Feinberg, *Social Philosophy* (Englewood Cliffs, New Jersey: Prentice-Hall, 1973), pp. 25-26.
3. Gerald Dworkin, "Paternalism," in Richard A. Wasserstrom (ed.), *Morality and the Law* (Belmont, Calif.: Wadsworth Publishing Company, 1971), pp. 107-126.
4. See Laurance T. Wren, "Status of the Law on Medical and Religious Conflicts in Blood Transfusions," in Samuel Gorovitz *et al.* (eds.), *Moral Problems in Medicine* (Englewood Cliffs, New Jersey: Prentice-Hall, 1976), pp. 234-238.
5. Robert M. Veatch, *Death, Dying, and the Biological Revolution* (New Haven, Conn.: Yale University Press, 1976), p. 117.
6. A recent medical development has added a new twist to the question of blood transfusions for Jehovah's Witnesses. A fluorocarbon mixture called Fluosol is now being used as a blood substitute. Fluosol can carry vast amounts of oxygen and do the work of blood until the patient's body has replenished its own supply. Jehovah's Witnesses apparently have no objections to the use of artificial blood and there have been several cases where this treatment has been successful. See *Time*, December 3, 1979, p. 90.
7. Quoted in George Thomas, Robert W. Edmark, and Thomas Jones, "Issues Involved with Surgery on Jehovah's Witnesses," in *Moral Problems in Medicine*, p. 240.
8. Veatch, *Death, Dying, and the Biological Revolution*, p. 119.
9. The cases that I mention here are discussed by Veatch, *Death, Dying, and the Biological Revolution*, pp. 125-127.
10. See Veatch's discussion in *Death, Dying, and the Biological Revolution*, pp. 136-137.
11. See Robert C. Underwood, "*In re* Brooks Estate," in *Moral Problems in Medicine*, pp. 232-234. See also, Veatch, *Death, Dying, and the Biological Revolution*, p. 154.
12. For a discussion of Muir's ruling, the reversal by the Supreme Court of New Jersey, and a comparison of the Heston and Quinlan cases, see Veatch, *Death, Dying, and the Biological Revolution*, pp. 136-144.
13. Here I borrow from the extensive discussion by Veatch, *Death, Dying, and the Biological Revolution*, pp. 133-136.
14. Veatch, *Death, Dying, and the Biological Revolution*, p. 135.
15. This case is presented by Robert M. Veatch, *Case Studies in Medical Ethics*, pp. 315-316.
16. For a discussion of this topic, see Veatch, *Death, Dying, and the Biological Revolution*, pp. 129-131.

17. J. Skelly Wright, "Application of President and Directors of Georgetown College," in *Moral Problems in Medicine*, p. 231.
18. Quoted in Veatch, *Death, Dying, and the Biological Revolution*, p. 156.
19. For a brief discussion of this case see Veatch, *Death, Dying, and the Biological Revolution*, pp. 157-158. See also, Wren, "Status of the Law on Medical and Religious Conflicts in Blood Transfusions," p. 237.
20. For an extensive discussion of this, see Veatch, *Death, Dying, and the Biological Revolution*, pp. 159-161.
21. The remaining part of this chapter has been previously published as "Treatment Without Consent," in James B. Wilbur (ed.), *The Life Sciences and Human Values: Proceedings of the Thirteenth Conference on Value Inquiry* (State University of New York at Geneseo, 1979), pp. 159-172.
22. These codes are reprinted in the Appendix.
23. Veatch, *Death, Dying, and the Biological Revolution*, pp. 121-122.
24. See Ruth Faden and Alan Faden, "False Belief and the Refusal of Medical Treatment," *Journal of Medical Ethics*, Vol. 3 (1977), pp. 133-136.
25. Faden and Faden, "False Belief and the Refusal of Medical Treatment," p. 134, argue that a physician does have an obligation to try to change a patient's false belief. They later argue (p. 135) that if the patient is competent, then there are reasons for not allowing paternalistic interference in the case of a false belief. However, the reasons they give are not thoroughly developed; and in any case one cannot say that there is a consensus on the matter.
26. Mill, *On Liberty*, p. 95.
27. Dworkin, "Paternalism," p. 122.
28. Dworkin, "Paternalism," p. 122.
29. Quoted in Veatch, *Death, Dying, and the Biological Revolution*, p. 156.
30. This distinction is made by Gerasimos Santas in "The Socratic Paradoxes," *The Philosophical Review*, Vol. LXXIII (1964), pp. 154-155.
31. See Mill, *On Liberty*, Chapter IV, especially pp. 74-75 and pp. 81-82.
32. Faden and Faden, in "False Belief and the Refusal of Medical Treatment," p. 135, offer the following as a reason for not allowing a paternalistic intervention in cases of false belief: "the acceptance of even limited paternalistic intervention opens a Pandora's box which could substantially threaten freedom." No further explanation of this claim is offered, but perhaps they have in mind considerations of the sort that are cited here.
33. See clause (3), *i* of the AMA Guidelines in the Appendix.
34. The case of Phillip Becker has been widely discussed. It was the subject of a story on the television program *60 Minutes* (1980) and was discussed by columnist George Will in *Newsweek* (April 14, 1980, p. 112).

# 4

# Experimentation
# and the Use of
# Human Subjects

Most medical workers, qua medical workers, have at least two roles to play. On the one hand, each medical worker is a therapist. As a therapist, the medical worker has an obligation to promote the health of his or her patient. On the other hand, most medical workers are involved in research as well. As a scientist, the medical worker is seeking to advance the growth of knowledge in his or her special area of interest or competence. That most medical workers play each of these two roles is clear; that doing so can lead to serious moral problems is perhaps less obvious. Playing these two different roles can lead to a problem of conflicting loyalties. What one ought to do as a scientist or researcher may conflict with what one ought to do as a therapist. Doing what will lead to advances in one's area of expertise may require that one violate one's obligation to the patient. Our point of departure regarding this problem will be to examine briefly what the various codes of ethics say concerning the use of human subjects in experiments.

## CODES OF ETHICS AND EXPERIMENTATION

Several professional codes of ethics address the issue of experimentation. The codes to be discussed here—the Nuremberg Code, the Declaration of Helsinki, and the American Medical Association Guidelines for Clinical Investigation—focus on the relationship between the permissibility of using human subjects in experiments and the nature of informed consent.[1]

## The Nuremberg Code

The Nuremberg Code was written and published in 1948. The first article of that code states: "The voluntary consent of the human subject is *absolutely* essential." And lest this be misconstrued, the meaning of this statement is spelled out in detail in the remaining part of the first article. The person being used as a research subject should have the legal capacity to give consent. The subject must be capable of exercising free power of choice, without intervention of any element of force, fraud, deceit, duress, constraint, or coercion. The person in question must have a sufficient knowledge of the nature of the experiment so that he or she can make an understanding and enlightened decision about participating in it. As a result, the nature, duration, and purpose of the experiment must be made known to the subject. The subject must be made aware of all inconveniences, hazards, and possible adverse effects on his or her health that might reasonably be expected as a result of participating in the experiment. It is the duty and responsibility of the person who initiates, directs, or engages in the experiment to ascertain the quality of the consent. Several points in the Nuremberg Code are noteworthy. First, the requirement for voluntary consent is absolute; the code allows for no exceptions here. Second, because the subject must have the legal capacity to give consent, apparently children may never be used as experimental subjects. Third, the code requires that the subject be well informed as to the nature and purposes of the experiment and any possible risks involved. The idea here, presumably, is to ensure that the consent is informed consent. Finally, this code, unlike others, does not distinguish between therapeutic and nontherapeutic experiments.

## The Declaration of Helsinki

The Declaration of Helsinki also provides medical workers engaged in research involving human subjects with some recommendations. This code was adopted by the 18th World Medical Assembly, Helsinki, Finland, 1964. It was revised by the 29th World Medical Assembly, Tokyo, Japan, 1975. The Declaration of Helsinki emphasizes the distinction between therapeutic and nontherapeutic experiments. A therapeutic experiment is one in which a physician uses a new procedure or drug or an untried technique for the sole purpose of helping his or her patient. Usually what occasions the need for a therapeutic experiment is either that the standard methods of treating the problem have proved to be inefficacious or that these methods will be too risky for the patient (perhaps because of some other medical problem). If an experiment is therapeutic, then any advance in scientific knowledge as a result of it will be incidental. A nontherapeutic experiment is one in which the primary aim is to gain scientific knowledge. The subjects involved in a nontherapeutic experiment are not expected to benefit directly from it. The guidelines that should be followed in using human beings as experimental subjects differ depending on whether the experiment is therapeutic or nontherapeutic. It is also noted in the declaration that it is essential for the growth of medical knowledge that experiments be applied to humans.

Concerning therapeutic research, the following are some of the points made by the Declaration of Helsinki. (i) In treating a patient the physician must be free to use new therapeutic measures if in his or her judgment doing so offers hope of saving life, reestablishing health, or alleviating suffering. (ii) If at all possible, the physician should obtain the patient's freely given and fully informed consent. If the patient is legally incompetent, then consent should be obtained from the legal guardian. (iii) The physician may combine clinical research with professional care only to the extent that the clinical research is justified by its expected therapeutic value for the patient. In other words, a doctor may use his or her subject in an experiment only if it is reasonable to expect that there will be direct benefits for the patient-subject. The authors of this code obviously realize the dangers involved if a physician uses his or her own patients as subjects in an experiment. Thus they require that it be expected that the patient will directly benefit from the experiment. In short, this suggests that a medical worker may not use his or her patients as subjects in a nontherapeutic experiment. Whether the authors intended this to follow from their guidelines is not clear. It is clear, though, that they were especially concerned about a physician using his or her own patients as subjects. Obviously there are great dangers of subtle pressure and coercion here. To guard against this, they included the following:

"When obtaining informed consent for the research project the doctor should be particularly cautious if the subject is in a dependent relationship to him or her or may consent under duress. In that case the informed consent should be obtained by a doctor who is not engaged in the investigations and who is completely independent of this official relationship."

Concerning nontherapeutic experimentation, the following are some of the Declaration's recommendations. (Some of these points apply to therapeutic experiments as well.) (i) The nature, purpose, and potential risk of the experiment must be explained to the subject by the physician. (ii) At all times during the experiment the physician must be the protector of life and health of the person on whom research is being carried out. If the life or well-being of a human subject is threatened, the experiment must be stopped. (iii) The freely given and fully informed consent of the subject is necessary. If the person in question is legally incompetent, then the consent of the legal guardian must be procured. (iv) It is preferable that the consent be obtained in writing. (v) The subject or guardian must be free to withdraw from the experiment at any time.

It might be briefly noted how the Declaration of Helsinki differs from the Nuremberg Code. First, it does draw the distinction between therapeutic and nontherapeutic experiments. Second, it suggests that it is appropriate for the physician to take more liberties regarding the former than the latter. In particular, in some cases a therapeutic experiment may be performed without the consent of the patient. Finally, unlike the Nuremberg Code, the Declaration of Helsinki allows that incompetents may be used in nontherapeutic experiments if the consent of the legal guardian is obtained.

## American Medical Association Ethical Guidelines for Clinical Investigation

In 1966 the American Medical Association Ethical Guidelines for Clinical Investigation were issued. Like the Declaration of Helsinki, these guidelines distinguish between "clinical investigation primarily for treatment" and "clinical investigation primarily for the accumulation of scientific knowledge." Again, the restrictions on using human subjects differ in these two cases. Concerning therapeutic experimentation, the AMA Guidelines include the following provisions. (i) Normally voluntary consent must be obtained from the patient after the physician has indicated that he or she plans to use an investigational drug or experimental procedure. The physician should provide a reasonable explanation of the nature of the drug or procedure to be used. The physician should explain about the possible risks involved and the likely therapeutic benefits, and should answer any questions that the patient might have. (ii) However, if the physician judges that disclosure of such information would be expected to affect adversely the health of the patient or would be detrimental to the patient's best interests, such information may be withheld. (iii) Whenever emergency treatment is necessary and the patient is incapable of giving consent and no one is available who has the authority to act on the patient's behalf, consent may be assumed.

Concerning investigation which is primarily for the accumulation of scientifc knowledge, the AMA Guidelines are almost exactly like the Declaration of Helsinki. There is one important difference, however. It concerns the use of minors and mentally incompetent adults in nontherapeutic experiments. The Declaration of Helsinki merely requires that the consent of the legal guardian be obtained. The AMA Guidelines, however, have a special clause dealing with this case. The AMA Guidelines do require that the freely given and fully informed consent of the legal guardian be obtained before a minor or mentally incompetent person may be used as a subject in a nontherapeutic experiment. But a second condition must be satisfied as well. "The nature of the investigation is such that mentally competent adults would not be suitable subjects." When might it be the case that a competent adult would not be a suitable subject in an experiment? If the investigation is directed specifically at a medical problem that only children have or that only mentally retarded persons have, then it may well be the case that in order to make progress on the treatment of that problem, children or mentally retarded persons must be used as subjects in an experiment.

In summary, then, the Nuremberg Code allows no experimentation without the consent of the subject-patient; the Declaration of Helsinki allows for therapeutic experiments without consent only if it is not possible to obtain the patient's consent; the AMA Guidelines permit therapeutic experiments without consent only if the physician judges that seeking consent will be contrary to the patient's best interests or if the situation is such that the patient cannot speak for himself or herself. Concerning the use of children or the mentally incompetent as experimental subjects, the Nuremberg Code absolutely forbids it; the Declaration of Helsinki allows it if the legal guardian has consented; and the AMA Guidelines permit their use only if the guardian has consented and a competent adult could not serve as a suitable subject in the experiment. In all cases, the Nuremberg Code is the most restrictive. Concerning the appropriateness of therapeutic experimentation, the AMA Guidelines are less restrictive than the Declaration of Helsinki in that only the former seems to allow for paternalistic treatment without consent when obtaining consent would be possible. Regarding the use of children or the mentally incompetent in nontherapeutic experiments, the Declaration of Helsinki is less restrictive than the AMA Guidelines.

## THE MORAL ISSUES

What are the moral questions concerning the use of human beings as experimental subjects? Most of the issues center around the notion of consent. Three questions seem of upmost importance here. (i) Did the person consent to being used as an experimental subject? (ii) If so, was the consent freely given? (iii) If so, was it fully informed consent? If the answer to any of these questions is "no," then serious moral questions are raised about the appropriateness of the experiment in question. If the answer to all three questions is "yes" and if the subjects are legally competent, then it is usually assumed that there are no moral objections to the arrangement. One possible exception arises, however, if the experiment involves overwhelming risks to the human subjects. It might be suggested that in cases like this using people as subjects is wrong even if they consent. Of course, to forbid the use of humans in such a case is paternalistic, but some have thought, perhaps correctly, that it is a justified instance of paternalism.

It seems quite reasonable to say that in emergency cases, situations in which the patient is unable to speak for himself or herself, therapeutic experimentation is morally justified (assuming that the medical evidence warrants it). When the patient is able to speak for himself or herself, then therapeutic experimentation without consent is just a specific case of treatment without consent. In the case of therapeutic experiments, as well as that of normal treatment, it can be argued that the requirement that the patient consent is virtually absolute, though, as indicated earlier, doubts can arise when the treatment in question involves the simple running of a test. Since this ground has already been covered, let us focus on the question of whether nontherapeutic experimentation without consent is ever justified.

Why might someone think that it would be appropriate to conduct a nontherapeutic experiment on human beings without their consent? Clearly in some cases if the subjects knew about the nature of the experiment it would seriously jeopardize the results. Certainly this is true in the case of experiments involving the use of placebos. The usual argument to justify nontherapeutic experiments without the consent of the subjects is a utilitarian one; that is, it is an argument that appeals to the good consequences of such experiments in certain circumstances. It is claimed that if the following conditions obtain, then there are strong utilitarian reasons for experimenting without the consent of the subjects: (1) there is no serious threat of harm to the subjects; (2) considerable benefits may be accrued from the experiment, for example, the growth of scientific knowledge, the development of cures for future patients, and the like; and (3) these benefits cannot be achieved if consent is required. The idea here is simple enough. There are certain highly desirable benefits that can be achieved only if human subjects are used in experiments without their consent. And since it is very unlikely that these subjects will be harmed, it is appropriate to use them without their consent.

Before discussing the argument that nontherapeutic experiments without consent are always unjustified, it is worth noting that a very similar argument is used to support therapeutic experiments without the patient's consent. This argument is also utilitarian in nature, but might be called the paternalistic argument. It is an argument used to justify the position supported by the AMA Guidelines that a physician may use a therapeutic experimental procedure without the consent of the patient if he or she believes that the knowledge would be detrimental to the patient's best interests. In effect, this argument states that therapeutic experimentation without consent is justified if the following two conditions obtain: (1) the new procedure or experimental drug is more likely to benefit the patient than any other procedure or drug available; and (2) these benefits cannot be achieved if the consent of the patient is required. Although the case for therapeutic experimentation without consent will not be discussed here, it is worth noting that someone might raise the following objection. The AMA Guidelines, a critic might argue, seem to approve of the paternalistic argument sketched here. Yet when the analogous version of this argument is applied to the case of nontherapeutic experiments without consent, it seems to be rejected. Aren't the authors of the AMA Guidelines being inconsistent? The appropriate response is that they are not being inconsistent. In the case of the paternalistic argument, an individual is being forced to benefit himself or herself; in the case of the utilitarian argument, an individual is being forced to benefit others. Even the staunchest opponents of paternalism are usually willing to concede that forcing an individual to benefit others is a more serious infringement of liberty than forcing an individual to benefit himself or herself. Thus the AMA position is not inconsistent, as a critic might charge.

To return to nontherapeutic experiments without consent, many will argue that they are never justified. Such persons usually claim that the right to self-determination is violated when experiments of this sort are conducted. A person has the right to be autonomous, and this includes the right not to be manipulated against his or her will. If a person is used as an experimental subject without his or her consent, then clearly this is a case of manipulation. And, the argument usually concludes, the right to self-determination cannot be overridden by utilitarian considerations. This argument, of course, is a deonotological one. In comparing the utlitarian and deontological arguments on this issue, it may be difficult to decide between them in the abstract. It will be helpful, then, to examine two case studies where these arguments have actually emerged.

## TWO CASE STUDIES

### The Jewish Chronic Disease Hospital Case

This case occurred at the Jewish Chronic Disease Hospital in New York City.[2] It drew a lot of publicity early in 1964 because it appeared to be a case of a nontherapeutic experiment done without the informed consent of the subjects. The case involved two doctors, Emanuel Mandel, the medical director of the Chronic Disease Hospital, and Chester Southam, the person directing the research in question. Southam was involved in a research project in which live cancer cells were being injected into hospitalized patients. His work at the Chronic Disease Hospital involved 22 seriously ill and debilitated patients. The research in question involved a study in cancer immunology. Within the scientific community the research was thought to be important.

Southam, upon receiving Mandel's approval, conducted one phase of his research on the 22 patients in the Chronic Disease Hospital. Southam's work involved the injection of tissue-cultured cancer cells into human subjects. His goal was to determine the speed with which the injected substance was rejected by the body. Earlier phases of his research had demonstrated that healthy persons reject the tissue-culture in four to six weeks, but that persons already ill with advanced cancer took a longer time to reject them, usually two to three months. Southam wanted to explain this slower rejection rate. He hypothesized that the slower rate of rejection in the cancer patients was attributable to the fact that they had cancer. He realized, however, that another hypothesis seemed equally plausible: namely, that the slower rate of rejection was due to the general debility that accompanies any chronic illness. In order to confirm his own hypothesis, Southam needed to conduct an experiment on patients severely ill with nonmalignant diseases. Thus he secured an agreement from Mandel to collaborate on such an experiment. They selected 22 patients from the Jewish Chronic

Disease Hospital. Three of these patients had cancer and were used as controls. The other 19 had a chronic, nonmalignant illness. Each of the patient-subjects was asked if he or she would consent to an injection which was described as a test to discover resistance or immunity to disease. They were told, correctly, that a lump would form and that in a few weeks it would go away. They were not told that this procedure was unrelated to their own condition, nor were they told that the substances to be injected consisted of live cancer cells. According to the record all of the patients agreed to the injection and none suffered any ill effects.

Southam and Mandel were heavily criticized for this experiment. The case received so much publicity that the Division of Professional Conduct of the State of New York had to deal with it. The Regents of the University of the State of New York had to investigate the case, since they were responsible for licensing the medical profession. The charges against the two doctors were "unprofessional conduct" and "fraud and deceit in the practice of medicine." The critics charged that Southam and Mandel took advantage of the chronically ill patients.

Southam and Mandel offered a spirited defense of their actions. The first point that they made was that the experiments involved no harm or risk to the subjects involved. This, of course, was correct. Nevertheless the regents wanted to know why the subjects were not fully informed about the nature of the procedure. In particular, they were not told that they were being injected with cancer cells. The reason that the word "cancer" was not used, the physicians claimed, was that this information was not pertinent to the experience the subjects would have. Moreover, the word "cancer" has a tremendous emotional disvalue. Most prospective subjects would experience an unwarranted and irrational fear upon hearing that cancer cells were to be injected into their bodies. In other words, there were benefits that could come from the experiment; there was no threat of harm to the subjects; and these benefits could not be achieved if the subjects were fully informed (because they would irrationally refuse to consent).

A second point made by the defendants was that the consent of the patient-subjects had been obtained. They had asked the subjects before injecting the cells, and each had given his consent. What was at issue, though, was the quality of this consent. Thirdly, Southam and Mandel claimed that the patients benefited from this experiment. Because they were subjects in the experiment, these patients received more attention and naturally this improved the care they received. Fourthly, the lawyers for these physicians argued that at the time of their actions there were no clear-cut medical or professional standards which they violated. As a result, it was claimed, if they were found guilty and punished, this would amount to *ex post facto* legislation. Finally, their lawyers argued, many other members of the medical profession followed the same sort of practices and procedures that Southam and Mandel had followed. If this conduct were widespread within the profession, it could not be "unprofessional," they reasoned.

In spite of this defense, the regents decided against the two doctors. However, the penalty meted out was very light. Their licenses were suspended for one year, but the execution of the sentences was stayed. As a result, they were put on probation for one year and permitted to continue to practice medicine. Nevertheless the points raised by the regents against the doctors are important. First, it was judged that the experiment was nontherapeutic. Southam and Mandel had maintained that the subjects stood to benefit because they would receive more attention and closer care. The regents argued, however, that these benefits were incidental and unrelated to the nature of the experiment. The remote possibility that the subjects might benefit because they are taking part in the experiment does not make it a therapeutic one. To be therapeutic, an experiment must have as its principal aim the benefit of the patient-subjects involved. This is an important point because if the broader notion of "therapeutic" were accepted, practically every experiment would be therapeutic and the point of the distinction would be lost. Surely the regents were correct in ruling that this research was not therapeutic.

Secondly, it was judged that the consent in question was not sufficient. The subjects were not given all of the information, and so their consent was not fully informed. Of course, Southam and Mandel argued that the information they withheld from the subjects was not needed in order for them to make a rational decision. The regents countered, however, that it is the subject who has the right to decide what factors are relevant to his or her consent, regardless of whether anyone else thinks it is relevant to take those factors into account. The subject has a right to know all of the material facts and he or she may refuse to participate for any reason whatsoever. Even if the experiment will benefit some and harm no one, fully informed consent is necessary. We can see, then, that the regents reject the utilitarian argument and accept instead the appeal to the right to self-determination. It is not unreasonable to construe them as saying that in this case the subjects were unfairly manipulated by the researchers. In effect, the position of the regents is that in a nontherapeutic experiment the deliberate non-disclosure of material facts is not different than deliberate misrepresentation of such facts. This second point is important and quite plausible.[3] Finally, the regents claimed that in some cases the subjects in question were incapable of giving consent. This was because in some cases the subjects were surely not competent and were not capable of understanding the nature of the experiment to which they were consenting.

The dispute concerning the permissibility of this particular experiment brings out the standard utilitarian and deontological arguments. There are, of course, other complicating factors. One concerns whether the experiment was therapeutic or nontherapeutic. On this issue, the position of the regents seems far more plausible. The more general question, though, of whether a nontherapeutic experiment of this sort (one in which fully informed consent is missing) is permissible will be left for the reader to decide. The hope is that this case and the one that follows will enable you to see more clearly the importance of the differences between the utilitarian and deontological arguments on the issue of nontherapeutic experiments without consent.

## The Willowbrook State Hospital Case

Willowbrook State Hospital is an institution on Staten Island, New York, which treats mentally retarded children.[4] In 1949 the population of Willowbrook was approximately 200. In 1972 there were 5200 residents, 3800 of whom were severely retarded. In 1949 hepatitis was detected among some of the residents of Willowbrook. In 1954 Dr. Saul Krugman was appointed as a consultant in pediatrics and in infectious diseases. He discovered that a number of infectious diseases were prevalent at Willowbrook; included among them were hepatitis, measles, shigellosis, parasitic infections, and respiratory infections. Dr. Krugman and his associates, Drs. Joan Giles and Jack Hammond, began studies on hepatitis. Because many of the severely retarded children were not toilet-trained and because infectious hepatitis is transmitted by way of the intestinal-oral route, nearly all suspectible children admitted to Willowbrook became infected within the first year. Between 1956 and 1970, 10,000 children were admitted to the Willowbrook Hospital. Of those, 750–800 were admitted to the research unit of Krugman, Giles, and Hammond. The researchers injected these children-subjects with infected serum to produce in them the strain of hepatitis already prevalent at Willowbrook. The researchers hoped to gain a better understanding of hepatitis and to develop some methods of immunizing against it. Only children whose parents gave written consent were used as subjects.

In the early 1970s this experiment was widely and critically discussed. Drs. Krugman, Giles, and Hammond, however, defended the experiment; they argued that no wrong was done. In particular, they made four points in their defense. First, the researchers argued that the children used as subjects were not harmed; or at least they were not made worse off than they would have been in the natural conditions existing at Willowbrook. Secondly, it was claimed that in some respects the children benefited. Because they were being admitted to a special, well-equipped, and well-staffed unit, they would be isolated from the other infectious diseases so prevalent at Willowbrook. Moreover, since contracting hepatitis was more or less inevitable for a child at Willowbrook, it would be better to get the disease under these highly controlled conditions. Thirdly, the children used as subjects were likly to have a subclinical infection (one not easily detected, which precedes the appearance of typical symptoms of a disease) followed by immunity to the particular hepatitis virus. And finally, they argued, the only children used were those whose parents gave informed consent. One can see that the classical utilitarian elements are present in the defense offered by Krugman, Giles, and Hammond. They wanted to emphasize that the children were made no worse off, that in fact they were benefited, that society might benefit (from the growth of knowledge), and that the fully informed consent of the parents was given. Like the researchers involved in the Jewish Chronic Disease Hospital case, these scientists tried to argue, in effect, that the experiment was therapeutic in nature and that consent had been obtained. The utilitarian considerations served as backup. Obviously it is more difficult to justify a nontherapeutic experiment without consent than any other, so it is not surprising that the doctors denied that they were engaged in such an experiment.

Many people in the medical community were outraged upon learning about the nature of this experiment.[5] Many objections were raised about the nature of this experiment and the major ones were the following. First, some argued that mentally retarded persons should never be used as experimental subjects, especially mentally retarded children. Such children are at a distinct disadvantage; they are unable to speak for or defend themselves. As a result, the possibility of abuse is much greater in these cases than when competent adults are used as subjects. And, some critics argued, even if the parents did consent, that does not justify the use of mentally retarded children. Clearly in these experiments on hepatitis, competent adults could have served as suitable subjects. It appears that mentally retarded children were used merely because they were convenient. Second, some have charged that though the parents of the children did consent, their consent was not freely given. It was coerced or pressured, if you will.[6] It was charged that in the later years when parents applied for their children to be admitted to Willowbrook, they received a form letter stating that no space was available. Shortly thereafter the parents would receive a letter saying that there were few spaces available in the hepatitis unit. So if the parents were willing to consent to research upon their children, they would be admitted to Willowbrook; otherwise, not. Clearly this put the parents in an untenable position; in order to receive institutionalization for their severely retarded child, they had to consent to allowing him or her to be used as an experimental subject.

A third objection to this experiment is that it was in no way therapeutic. Any benefits that the children-subjects might receive—such as isolation from the other infectious diseases—were clearly incidental. In no way was the chief aim of this experiment to benefit the children used as subjects. Furthermore, many claimed that the possible benefits to the institution or to society from this experiment were minimal. These researchers claimed that from these studies they hoped to learn how to control the outbreak of hepatitis in the institution. Some critics have charged, however, that the aim was much less noble. Paul Ramsey, for example, has argued that the experiments were merely designed to duplicate and confirm the efficacy of gamma globulin in immunization against hepatitis. What the researchers really wanted to do, he argues, was simply to develop further and improve upon that inoculum.[7] Of course, even if Ramsey is right, these goals may be worth pursuing. An advocate of the utilitarian argument may have no problem admitting this. However, the experiment would be easier to justify (from a utilitarian point of view) if the work were more original and of a groundbreaking nature.

There are also serious moral questions raised because these researchers withheld from the general population at Willowbrook an inoculation known to have some degree of efficacy. This is a fourth objection that has been raised concerning this experiment.[8] Surely it was known by the researchers that those from whom the gamma globulin was withheld were in more danger than the experimental subjects. It seems that those who were part of the general population at Willowbrook were being treated as a means only. They were unnecessarily being placed in a situation that was more risky than need be. This raises a serious moral question that those engaged in medical research cannot help but face. In order to confirm that a given treatment is efficacious, one needs a control group from whom the treatment is withheld. But sometimes it seems unfair to withhold such treatment, especially if it is quite reasonable to believe (perhaps because of experiments done on animals) that the treatment will be effective.

A situation like this occurred in 1960 with the development of the polio vaccine.[9] Drs. Weller, Enders, and Robbins had what they thought was an effective vaccine. But in order to satisfy the demands of scientific rigor, they needed a group from whom the vaccine was withheld. Thus approximately thirty thousand children were injected with a substance which was known to be useless in the prevention of polio. It was known, of course, that some of these children would get polio and die from it, but this seemed to be the only way to confirm that their vaccine was effective. It is worth noting that the justification for such an act is utilitarian, but in this case there clearly is risk for the nonconsenting human subjects. Another case like this has occurred much more recently. It was discovered that a drug, sulfinpyrazone, used for years to relieve gout seemed to reduce significantly the risk of death from a second heart attack.[10] The drug appears to be so effective that it would be unfair to keep it from any heart-attack victims; but unless it is kept from some of these victims, confirming its usefulness will remain impossible. The case at Willowbrook may have been unlike the two just described. When the conditions present in the latter two cases obtain, however, the issue is a very difficult one.

Let us consider another objection that has been raised against the experiment at Willowbrook. As part of their defense, Krugman, Giles and Hammond claimed that the children used as subjects actually benefited. And it seems clear that their claim is correct. The children who were subjects did receive more attention and were protected from the other contagious diseases that were prevalent at Willowbrook. But why did they benefit? It is clear that the only reason that they benefited was that the normal conditions at Willowbrook were so horrendous that almost anything would be an improvement. Thus the claim that the subjects benefited seems somewhat tainted. It seems that the experimenters took advantage of them because of the terrible conditions they endured. What they should do, it can be argued, is to improve these conditions. One critic puts it this way: "The duty of a pediatrician in a situation such as exists at Willowbrook State School is to attempt to improve that situation, not to turn it to his advantage for experimental purposes, however lofty the aims."[11] Thus, the critic would contend, these doctors should have been addressing themselves to the fundamental problem of why infectious diseases were so prevalent at Willowbrook.

This last objection raises the more general issue of what obligations a person has in situations that are less than ideal. It is controversial because there are at least two different positions that can be taken on this issue.[12] The view of the critic is a morally rigorous position, one an idealist might adopt. Advocates of this position argue that the moral duty of any researcher encountering conditions as bad as those at Willowbrook is to improve those conditions rather than take advantage of them. Perhaps not everyone has an obligation to be beneficent. But when a person has the skills necessary to improve those conditions and when that person has a special relationship with the potential subjects (as the researchers at Willowbrook did have with the children), then surely there is an obligation to alleviate those fundamental problems. Thus a researcher should never take advantage of those who find themselves in poor social conditions; rather he or she should work to alter the situation.

Those inclined to defend the researchers at Willowbrook (at least against this objection) will take what might be called the utilitarian position on this issue. According to the utilitarian position, it is unrealistic to require researchers to try to change all of the bad social conditions that they might encounter. What they should do instead is to make the best of a bad situation. We may lament the fact that some are so bad off that they might actually benefit by becoming a subject in an experiment like that conducted at Willowbrook, but one cannot expect researchers to change the world overnight. In such situations it is appropriate, then, to make a trade, as it were. A person will be given certain "benefits" if he or she grants to the researcher the privilege of using him or her as an experimental subject. And it is worth noting here that the benefits in question need not be medical ones, though they were at Willowbrook. In the past prisoners would volunteer for experiments in order to receive the benefits of $1 a day or some extra cigarettes. Clearly such "rewards" are perceived as benefits only because prisoners have no other means of earning any money. Thus the researcher would be taking advantage of their bad situation. But is this an impermissible trade off?

It might be noted in conclusion that some will object to the Willowbrook experiment simply because children were used as experimental subjects. Certainly suspicions about using children in experiments are common and with good reason. Unlike adults, many children are not able to speak for themselves or to understand what is in their best interests. Moreover, since many of the capacities that children have are undeveloped, it seems that the risks involved in using them as subjects are greater. The chance that they will suffer irreparable harm seems greater than in the case of adults. Worries about the possibilities of psychological harm that might be done to the child-subject are also common. But to advocate an absolute prohibition on the use of children as experimental subjects seems to go too far. There are biological differences between children and adults, differences in anatomy, metabolism, and the like. And one would expect that certain drugs would produce different effects in children than adults. In addition, children are subject to some diseases not prevalent among adults. Thus, it would seem that if any advances in treating children are to be made they must sometimes be used in experiments. This explains the rationale underlying the pronouncement in the AMA Ethical Guidelines for Clinical Investigation concerning the use of children as subjects. The guidelines do not absolutely prohibit the use of children, but before they may be used it must be the case that adults could not serve as suitable subjects. Given our hesitancy about using children and yet given the obvious need to use them sometimes, the position taken in the AMA Guidelines seems quite plausible. At any rate, to object to the Willowbrook experiment on the general grounds that children should never be used as experimental subjects seems unrealistic.

## CONCLUSIONS

The reason for examining these two case studies was to elucidate concrete examples of apparently nontherapeutic experiments. Thus would better enable us to choose between the utilitarian and deontological positions on the question of whether nontherapeutic experiments without consent are ever permissible. Certainly in these two cases the permissibility of the experiments seems doubtful. However, it may not be justifiable to infer from this that no nontherapeutic experiment without consent is permissible. Two examples are not enough to justify such a general conclusion. Examining these cases should help us to see what moral problems emerge in discussing nontherapeutic experiments without consent. Whether the absolute prohibition advocated by the defender of the deonotological position goes too far is perhaps best left to the reader to decide.

It is appropriate to end this chapter by mentioning briefly a case discussed by Robert Veatch.[13] The case in question involves the use of placebos, and such experiments will almost always be jeopardized if the consent of the subject is required. Several researchers were interested in testing psychoactive drugs. In doing so, they always had to use a control group to whom a placebo was given. These scientists were careful to explain the risks involved in these experiments and to obtain the consent of the subjects. There was one risk, however, that they could not explain. Some of the subjects would be receiving medication that was known to be ineffective. Yet if these subjects were told this, the experiment would be ruined. One of the researchers wanted to explain to all of the patients that some of them would be receiving placebos. The others, though, felt that even this information might cause some of the subjects to report inaccurately their perceptions. After discussion, the doctors decided to do an experiment to see what the effects are of telling a subject that he or she has a chance of receiving a placebo. Thus one group was told that each of them had one chance in four of receiving a placebo. This information was not given to the other group, though in fact each of them also had a one in four chance of receiving a placebo. Clearly, this is a nontherapeutic experiment. It is also plausible to say that the possible benefits of the experiment are great. If it were to turn out that telling subjects they had a chance of receiving a placebo did not affect the results of the experiment, all future researchers could obtain fully informed consent when conducting such experiments. Yet in this particular experiment consent cannot be obtained. The goal, after all, is to see if informing the subjects makes any difference.

These researchers face a difficult choice: either there is certain knowledge that may never justifiably be pursued or that knowledge can be sought only if human beings are used as subjects without their consent. Neither of these choices seems acceptable. It seems too extreme and stifling to say that certain knowledge may never be pursued. But our reticence to use people as experimental subjects without their explicit consent remains. Veatch offers a suggestion for avoiding this dilemma by appealing to the notion of "implied consent." "The implied consent of the real subjects may reasonably be assumed if, and only if, there is good evidence that a reasonable person would consent if he had been adequately informed."[14] And how does one tell if a reasonable person would consent? Veatch suggests that a mock subject group be selected from the same population as the real subjects. The nature, purpose, and possible risks of the experiment should be explained to this mock group and then they should be asked if they would consent to be a subject in such an experiment. If an overwhelming majority say that they would consent, then it can reasonably be assumed that the real subjects would consent too. This will allow us to pursue nontherapeutic experiments that are important and are such that consent cannot be obtained.

Veatch's proposal is interesting and thought provoking, but it will not be evaluated here. It is worth stressing, however, what motivates his suggestion. An absolute prohibition against nontherapeutic experiments without consent seems to go too far, but extreme caution must be followed when using people without their explicit approval.

## SUMMARY

The principal concern of this chapter has been the appropriateness of using human beings as subjects in nontherapeutic experiments. Many important questions were ignored. For example, is it permissible to use a human being as an experimental subject when he or she has given fully informed consent but when there is great risk involved? Instead the question of whether it is ever permissible to use human beings as experimental subjects when they have not consented and do not stand to benefit directly from the experiment was dealt with. The utilitarian position on this issue is that if there is no risk to the subject, if the potential benefits from the experiment are great, and if the benefits could not be obtained if consent were required, then nontherapeutic experiments without consent are justified. By contrast, some deontologists argue that a medical worker is never permitted to use a human being as an experimental subject without his or her consent. To do so is an inappropriate infringement on a person's freedom. Two case studies were presented to illustrate how each of these positions has emerged in practice. When examining these two positions, dissatisfaction arises: the utilitarian position seems to allow for too much experimentation without consent, but the deontological position seems too prohibitive: it puts forever out of our reach certain useful knowledge. This is an issue concerning which a compromise would be desirable. Robert Veatch has suggested such a proposal, and it was explained at the end of the chapter.

## CASE STUDY

The Food and Drug Administration (FDA) was asked recently to review a new drug called isoprinosine. It is thought that this drug will be effective in treating a form of encephalitis (inflammation of the brain) that is rare but fatal. Normally the FDA will not evaluate new drugs without placebo tests, tests in which the medication is withheld from a control group. Physicians have objected, however, that keeping a potentially life-prolonging drug from patients is wrong. To receive FDA approval, a new drug or medication must not only be harmless; it must also be proven effective. In the case of isoprinosine, the agency claimed that there was not enough evidence to prove that the drug was effective. They made this claim in spite of the fact that it has been used successfully in many nations, including England, France, and West Germany. In other words, clinical experience has suggested that the drug is effective, but no scientific tests have been done to prove it. To establish the scientific evidence, suppose that an experiment were set up. Ten persons with this rare form of encephalitis are recruited as subjects. Five are given isoprinosine, while five receive a treatment known to be not very effective.[15]

## Discussion Questions

1. Is this experiment therapeutic or nontherapeutic? In answering this, remember that there are two groups of subjects.
2. Would it be appropriate to conduct this experiment without the consent of the ten subjects? Would it be justifiable to conduct it if each of the subjects consented? What sort of difficulties would there be in getting the consent of the subjects? How would Robert Veatch's proposal concerning experimentation without consent work in this case?
3. Suppose that at some point in this experiment it became clear that the subjects receiving isoprinosine were benefiting greatly and that the other subjects were deteriorating. Would those conducting the experiment have an obligation to begin administering the isoprinosine to all of the subjects? If they did, would this affect the validity of the results?
4. It is the FDA's requirement of a medication's proven effectiveness that prevents such drugs as Laetrile (a drug claimed by some to be effective in fighting cancer) and DSMO (dimethyl sulfoxide, a drug claimed by some to be effective in reducing the pain and swelling of arthritis, among other things) from being made available to the public. On what sort of principle is the policy that a medication must be proven effective (and not merely harmless) before it can be made available to patients based? Do you agree with this policy?

## SUGGESTIONS FOR FURTHER READING

Alexander Morgan Capron, "Human Experimentation: Basic Issues," in Warren T. Reich (ed.), *Encyclopedia of Bioethics* (New York: The Free Press, 1978), pp. 692-698.
Charles Fried, "Human Experimentation: Philosophical Aspects," in Warren T. Reich (ed.), *Encyclopedia of Bioethics* (New York: The Free Press, 1978), PP. 699-702.
Franz J. Ingelfinger, "Informed (But Uneducated) Consent," in Thomas A. Mappes and Jane S. Zembaty (eds.), *Biomedical Ethics* (New York: McGraw-Hill Book Company, 1981), pp. 155-156.
Hans Jonas, "Philosophical Reflections on Experimenting with Human Subjects," in Thomas A. Mappes and Jane S. Zembaty (eds.), *Biomedical Ethics* (New York: McGraw-Hill Book Company, 1981), pp. 150-154.
Jessica Mitford, "Experimenting Behind Bars," in Samuel Gorovitz *et al.* (eds.), *Moral Problems in Medicine* (Englewood Cliffs, New Jersey: Prentice-Hall, 1976), pp. 162-167.
Paul Ramsey, *The Patient as Person* (New Haven, Conn.: Yale University Press, 1970), pp. 40-58.
Robert M. Veatch, *Case Studies in Medical Ethics* (Cambridge, Mass.: Harvard University Press, 1977), pp. 290-302.

## NOTES

1. These codes are reprinted in the Appendix.
2. In presenting this case I draw heavily from Elinor Langer's "Human Experimentation: New York Verdict Affirms Patient's Rights," *Science* 151: 11, pp. 663-666.
3. It must be noted, however, that requiring researchers to present any information to the subject that he or she might consider relevant can lead to absurdities in extreme cases. This point is made very sardonically by Preston J. Burnham in "Medical Experimentation on Humans," *Science* 152: 22, pp. 448-450.
4. This case is widely discussed in the literature on experimentation. I draw my presentation from Robert M. Veatch, *Case Studies in Medical Ethics* (Cambridge, Mass.: Harvard University Press, 1977), pp. 274-275; Tom L. Beauchamp and James F. Childress, *Principles of Biomedical Ethics* (New York: Oxford University Press, 1979), pp. 276-277; and Gorvitz *et al.* (eds.), *Moral Problems in Medicine* (Englewood Cliffs, N.J.: Prentice-Hall, 1976), pp. 123-129.
5. The criticisms of this experiment are far too numerous to list. I shall mention some of the more important ones in the text. These, as well as many others I do not mention, may be found in the following: "Letters: Experiments at the Willowbrook State School," in Samuel Gorovitz *et al.* (eds.), *Moral Problems in Medicine* (Englewood Cliffs, New Jersey: Prentice-Hall, 1976), pp. 126-129; Paul Ramsey, *The Patient as Person* (New Haven, Conn.: Yale University Press, 1970), pp. 47-58; and Veatch, *Case Studies in Medical Ethics*, pp. 274-277.

6.  See, for example, Ramsey, *The Patient as Person*, pp. 53–54.
7.  Ramsey, *The Patient as Person*, p. 47.
8.  Ramsey, *The Patient as Person*, p. 49.
9.  See Ronald Munson, "Medical Experimentation and Informed Consent," in Ronald Munson (ed.), *Intervention and Reflection* (Belmont, Calif.: Wadsworth Publishing, 1979), p. 224.
10. "Heart's Ease," *Newsweek*, February 20, 1978, p. 95.
11. Stephen Goldby, "Letters: Experimentation at the Willowbrook State School," in *Moral Problems in Medicine*, pp. 126–127.
12. These positions are discussed, though in a somewhat different way from my approach, by Veatch, *Case Studies in Medical Ethics*, p. 277.
13. Veatch, *Case Studies in Medical Ethics*, pp. 299–302.
14. Veatch, *Case Studies in Medical Ethics*, p. 302.
15. The controversy surrounding isoprinosine was reported in *Newsweek*, July 14, 1980. The experiment suggested here is hypothetical. As the article notes, the FDA has modified its position. In the case of isoprinosine, it still insists on controlled studies, but they need not involve a placebo.

# 5

# Killing,
# Letting Die,
# and
# Euthanasia

Euthanasia and abortion, the topics to be discussed in this and the next chapter, are called the life and death issues in medical ethics. Each issue has a social component and a private aspect. Because society has an interest in these matters, it is appropriate for legislators to pass laws dealing with them. Yet individual medical workers must make decisions about these issues quite apart from what the law says. If a woman requests an abortion, the physician must decide whether to comply or refuse. If a dying patient asks for a dosage of a lethal drug, the medical worker must decide whether to honor this request.

At stake in the issues of euthanasia and abortion is the value of life. Because most of us put a high value on life, any moral theory that fails to do so will seem implausible. There is at least a prima facie duty to preserve life. The interesting issue concerns when this duty may be overridden. Is it ever permissible not to preserve life? If so, when? In medical contexts, the claims that it is sometimes permissible not to preserve life and sometimes permissible to end life arise in the debates concerning euthanasia and abortion. In each of these cases some are tempted either not to save or actively to end the life of a being.

## THE MORAL STATUS OF ACTIONS

Since the preservation of life is a value of great significance, the factors which might affect the moral status of the act of ending life must be examined. Any given action has one of three moral statuses.[1] Some actions are *morally required*; that is, it would be wrong not to do those acts. Keeping a promise is an act that is (normally) required. Second, some actions are *merely permissible.*[2] To say that an act is merely permissible is to say that an agent may do or refrain from doing the act. With respect to merely permissible actions, a person is free to do as he or she wishes. Merely permissible acts are morally neutral. Examples of such actions include a decision to wear brown shoes, to eat cereal for breakfast, or to read Shakespeare instead of Dickens. The third moral status that an action might have is that of being *morally forbidden*. If an act is morally forbidden, then it is wrong to do that act. Uncontroversial examples of morally forbidden actions include killing, stealing, and torturing.

The moral status of actions is affected by the rights that beings have. Though no complete analysis of rights will be presented here, we can say that rights put legitimate restraints on how others may behave toward the being that possesses the rights. Rights generate obligations on others. That is, if a person has a right, then others have obligations with respect to that person. A distinction between positive and negative rights can be drawn, a distinction based on the difference between the sort of obligations others have. A positive right creates an obligation on others to perform a specific service for the person possessing the right. If $X$ has promised to help $Y$ this afternoon, then $Y$ has a positive right against $X$. $X$ has an obligation to serve $Y$ in the manner specified. The rights children have to be fed, clothed, and cared for by their parents are positive rights. By contrast, a negative right is a right to others' omissions or forbearances. For every negative right a person possesses, someone else has a duty to refrain from doing something. A person's property rights are negative; they impose on others the obligation not to take or use that property without the owner's permission. Similarly, the right not to be tortured is a negative right. As will be discussed later, there is some dispute about whether the right to life is a positive or a negative right.

## KILLING AND LETTING DIE

One factor relevant to the moral status of preserving life is the distinction between killing and letting die. Killing a being presumably involves a positive act that is the cause of that being's death. The locution "letting die" is ambiguous. It is sometimes said that a person let another being die when killing that being would also have been a plausible option. Suppose a person encounters a dying animal that is in severe pain and could be killed painlessly by being shot. If this person does not shoot the animal, it is said that he or she let it die. Often, though, the phrase "letting die" is used to indicate that a person refrained from saving a being. In this sense it cannot be said that a person let another die unless the following conditions are satisifed: (i) the person had the ability to save or to prolong the life of the one who died; (ii) the person had the opportunity to save or to prolong the life of the one who died; and (iii) the person knew that the first two conditions were satisfied. The reason for including these conditions is clear enough. If I cannot swim and have no other means available to save a drowning person, it is implausible to describe this as a case of my letting the person die. Similarly, if a person has a serious medical problem, which if not attended to will be fatal, it might be said plausibly that a physician present let the person die; but it would be ludicrous to say that a plumber (with no medical knowledge) let that person die. Lack of opportunity will also render the description "letting the person die" inaccurate. Even the best of swimmers cannot be said to have let a person drown if he or she is on the other side of a huge lake. And even if a person has the ability and opportunity to save another, it cannot be said that he or she has let that person die unless the person knew that he or she could have saved the other. Thus if I am a good swimmer and am in my oceanside home reading a philosophy book, I have both the ability and the opportunity to save the person drowning just outside my house. But if I do not know this, I cannot be said to have let the person die.

Not everyone agrees about the importance of the distinction between killing and letting die. With regard to this question there are two extreme theses, each of which has a number of advocates. The first thesis, thesis (I), is this: There is a morally relevant difference between killing and letting die, and that difference is such that killing is always worse, from the moral point of view, than letting die. Thesis (I) is widely accepted in the medical and legal communities, as will be seen when discussing the issue of euthanasia. Why would someone hold this position? Reasons to support the position are rarely articulated, but presumably the following considerations are what advocates of this view have in mind. Killing is a positive act that an agent performs; normally it brings about death sooner than it would otherwise occur. Letting die, by contrast, is merely refraining from acting. And, according to this view, a person is always more responsible for a positive act than for an ommission. So bringing about a death by killing is always worse than doing so by letting die. An example might be adduced to support this position. Suppose that you saw a man drowning but were unable (or unwilling) to save him. Wouldn't it be worse, from the moral point of view, for you to shoot the man rather than let him drown? Surely it would. To shoot him would preclude the possibility that he might be saved by someone else or by his own effort. So, it might be argued, thesis (I) is plausible.

Not all accept thesis (I), however. Some have argued for a second view, thesis (II): There is no morally relevant difference between killing and letting die; one is just as bad as the other. Reasons have been given to support this position. Its defenders argue that the two most important moral features, the result and the motive, are the same in cases of killing and letting die. The result is the death of a person, and the motive is apparently the desire for that death. (Recall that it cannot accurately be said that a person has let another die unless the person could have saved the other and knew this.) What else could be morally relevant? advocates of this view ask. Examples are often cited to lend credence to this position.[3] Suppose that Smith and Jones each stands to inherit a large sum of money from the death of his young son. Each devises a plan to kill his son and to make it look like an accident. Each decides to drown his boy while he is taking a bath. Smith carries out his plan according to schedule and thus can be said to have killed his son. Jones sets about to do the same. But just as he enters the bathroom, his son slips and hits his head, knocking him unconscious. Jones considers himself fortunate, noting that now he will not have to kill his son; he can simply let him die. Is the act of Jones less repugnant than that of Smith?—surely not. From the moral point of view, each has done the wrong thing. And this is so, even though it is true that Smith has killed his son and Jones has merely let his son die. So, the argument goes, there is no morally relevant difference between killing and letting die.

Each of theses (I) and (II) has a number of advocates. Yet neither of these views seems plausible. Many cases can be presented in which common sense tells us that letting die is worse than killing, thus casting doubt on thesis (I). Suppose that you come upon a car accident. The car has just burst into flames and a woman is trapped inside. It is apparent to you and to her that you will not be able to free her from the car. By now the fire is causing the woman great pain; few deaths are as excruciating as burning alive. You happen to have a gun with you and the woman begs you to shoot her. She cannot stand the pain any longer. Surely neither she nor we would accept it if you argued that you may not shoot her because killing is worse than letting die. In this case letting die is worse. Or consider this case. An infant is born severely deformed, so deformed that it cannot hope to live a satisfactory life, or even a life without great pain. It is decided by the parents and the doctor that in this case infant euthanasia is justified. The physician, however, believes that letting die is the only permissible form of euthanasia; killing is always wrong. So the physician instructs the nurses to cease all treatment and even to stop feeding the infant. Thus the infant is starved to death but not killed. Once it has been decided that the death of this infant is desirable, surely killing it painlessly is far preferable to letting it die of starvation. Clearly the latter sort of death is quite unpleasant. And suppose that a person found a severly injured animal that could not be saved but could be kept alive several more days in great pain. Certainly people's actual behavior in cases like this suggests that most believe killing in such a situation is far better than letting die. These examples, then, suggest that in at least some cases letting die is worse than killing. Thus thesis (I) seems dubious.

According to thesis (II) killing and letting die are not in themselves morally different. It can be noted immediately that the cases used against thesis (I) seem equally telling against thesis (II); if in some cases letting die is worse than killing, then there is sometimes a morally relevant difference. But there also seem to be some cases in which killing is worse than letting die. Consider the following two cases.[4] Suppose that six accident victims are brought to the emergency room. All six are near death, but one is much worse than the other five. The physician on duty judges correctly that there are two alternatives: the physician can devote all available time and resources to the one, thereby saving him or her but letting the other five die; or the physician can devote the necessary time and resources to the five at the expense of the one. But now consider another situation. Suppose that there are five moribund patients in the hospital. Each can be saved, however, if he or she receives an organ needed for transplantation. As it happens there is another patient in the hospital who has all of the organs needed by these patients and who is tissue compatible with each. Let us suppose further that the patient will die in nine months of an illness, but this disease does not adversely affect the needed organs. Again in this case a physician has two alternatives: to preserve the life of the one (for the remaining nine months) and let the five die; or to kill the one and use those organs to save the five. What should the physician do? Surely most people believe that killing the one is wrong. Forcing a patient to benefit others at the expense of his or her own life is not acceptable. And this is so even though death is imminent. But now notice the comparison of these two cases. In each case the physician could save five at the expense of one. And in each case the motive might have been the desire to save the greater number. Yet saving the greater number in the first case is permissible, but wrong in the second case. The most obvious difference in these two cases is that one is a case of letting a patient die to save five, while the other is a case of killing a patient to save five. If this is correct, further doubt has been cast on thesis (I).[5]

Each of the standard positions, thesis (I) and thesis (II), seems to be incorrect. If our judgments are reliable about these matters, it seems that sometimes killing is worse than letting die, sometimes letting die is worse than killing, and sometimes they are on a par. To say only this, however, leaves open many possibilities. For example, to say that killing is sometimes worse than letting die may mean that both are wrong but that killing is the graver wrong, or it may mean that in a given situation killing would be wrong but that letting die would be permissible. The same ambiguity is present when we say that letting die is sometimes worse than killing. And to assert that killing and letting die are sometimes on a moral par may mean that both are wrong or that both are justified. To sort through these complexities, one would like to have some principled way of determining whether killing or letting die is worse and whether either is permissible. To that end, let us examine a third thesis.

## THE DOCTRINE OF DOUBLE EFFECT

The doctrine of double effect is a principle that steers a course between theses (I) and (II) and which purports to provide guidance on these matters. Historically, the doctrine of double effect has its roots in Catholic theology. This doctrine yields judgments on the abortion issue that Catholic theologians find acceptable. But this principle can just as well be viewed as a competitor to theses (I) and (II). Before stating the doctrine, some terms, which are necessary to understand it, will be explained. The doctrine of double effect is based on a distinction between what a person foresees as a result of his or her action and what a person intends by such action. What is it that a person intends when he or she performs a voluntary action? According to this doctrine a person intends in the strictest sense only those things that he or she *aims at as ends* or those things aimed at as *direct means* to such ends. A consequence of a person's action which is known will occur, but which is neither the end sought nor the direct means to that end, is said to be merely foreseen. To illustrate, consider the following example. A patient has cancer. In the judgment of the physician, the treatment most likely to be successful is chemotherapy, and so that is what the physician recommends. The physician realizes that an unfortunate result of the chemotherapy is that the patient will become nauseous and lose hair. The end this doctor is aiming at is to help the patient. The means to this end is to initiate chemoterapy treatments. A foreseen but unintended consequence is that the patient will become nauseous and lose hair. This consequence is unintended in the technical sense because it is neither the end sought nor the direct means to that end. Intuitively it makes sense to say that this consequence is unintended because the physician in no way desires this end; if it were possible to administer the chemotherapy treatments without the accompanying nausea and hair loss, the physician would be delighted.

According to the doctrine of double effect a person is more responsible for what is intended as a result of a voluntary action than for what is merely foreseen will follow from such actions. Given these distinctions, the doctrine of double effect may now be stated as follows: It is permissible to bring about through voluntary actions an evil state of affairs just in case (i) the agent does not intend the evil that results and (ii) performing the action prevents a greater evil or the evil that does occur could only be prevented if the agent were to do evil intentionally. To explain briefly, clause (i) states that it is never permissible for a person, through voluntary actions, to bring about evil if that evil is the end sought or a direct means to that end. Clause (ii) appeals to a kind of proportionality. It states that even when the evil brought about is foreseen but unintended, it is permissible to allow it to occur only if doing so prevents a greater evil. This principle is called the doctrine of double effect because it distinguishes, for moral reasons, two different effects of an action: those aimed at or intended and those foreseen but in no way desired. The doctrine of double effect forbids a person to do evil intentionally. Bringing about an evil state of affairs is permitted only if the agent does not intend this.

Why should anyone accept this doctrine? One reason for doing so is that it yields intuitively plausible judgments in the cases examined above; it seems to avoid the pitfalls of theses (I) and (II). Consider the emergency case (discussed above) in which the physician has two choices: the physician may devote all available time and resources to one of six accident victims, thereby saving him or her but allowing the other five to die; or the physician may devote an equal amount of time and resources to each of the five, saving them but allowing the sixth to die. In this case the doctrine of double effect tells us that the physician may act to save the five. The end aimed at is to save five lives. The direct means to that end is to devote to each one-fifth of the physician's time and resources. The evil state of affairs that will result from this is that the sixth patient will die, but that this will occur is foreseen but unintended. Moreover, allowing this undesirable state of affairs to occur does prevent a greater evil, namely, the deaths of five patients. Thus the doctrine of double effect permits such an action. Now consider again the case of the five patients, each of whom needs an organ for transplantation. Another person in the hospital has each of the needed organs and is tissue compatible with each of the five. The doctrine of double effect does not permit us to kill the sixth person and to distribute his or her organs to the other five. The end aimed at is acceptable—to save five patients. However, the means to that end is to kill the one, and so this end can be achieved only by doing evil intentionally, something that the doctrine of double effect forbids. This principle, then, does yield plausible results in these two cases.

As noted earlier, Catholic theologians have accepted the doctrine of double effect because it, coupled with certain assumptions, supports a very conservative position on the abortion issue. Suppose that a woman is pregnant but that carrying the child full term will be very dangerous to her health; it is judged that she will probably die unless she obtains an abortion. (It must be supposed further, though this is often not pointed out, that ending the life of the fetus is evil in itself.) Abortion, even in this extreme case, is not permitted according to advocates of the doctrine of double effect (who accept the additional assumption). The end sought is to save the life of the woman. The direct means to that end, however, is to kill the fetus, and this is doing evil intentionally (granting that the fetus has the right to life). But isn't allowing the woman to die wrong too? It is not, according to the doctrine of double effect. The end sought is to save the child. The means to that end is to have the woman carry it full term. A foreseen but unintended consequence is that the woman will die. Thus the evil state of affairs brought about is unintended. If it is granted that the fetus has the right to life, then having the woman carry it full term does prevent an evil. And though it is not obvious that the evil it prevents is a greater evil (isn't the death of the woman at least as great an evil?), nevertheless this evil must be tolerated because the other evil—the woman's death—can be prevented only by intentionally doing evil. Thus a very conservative position on the abortion issue is maintained. Of course, this same conclusion might be embraced without adopting the doctrine of double effect. But that is not the point. The point is that one way of defending this position is by appealing to the doctrine of double effect (and the supplementary assumption).

Is the doctrine of double effect a plausible view? Many think not. Some reject the doctrine because of the conclusion drawn on the abortion issue by some of its defenders. This, however, is not a good reason for rejecting the doctrine of double effect. This doctrine does not force a person to adopt the position of the extreme conservative on the abortion issue unless additional assumptions about the nature of the fetus and the rights it possesses are made. And if these additional assumptions are made the doctrine of double effect need not be embraced in order to arrive at the conservative position. It would be better, then, to focus on more general objections raised against the doctrine of double effect. It must be admitted that the doctrine appears suspicious. It is far from obvious that so much should depend on whether a consequence was intended or merely foreseen, and it is natural to have an uneasy feeling about this doctrine. This uneasy feeling can be given more content. As a criticism of the doctrine of double effect, the following might be suggested: Through verbal manipulation the doctrine of double effect can be used to justify almost any conclusion wished for.[6] To support this criticism, the following case has been cited. Suppose that a group of ten people are exploring in a cave near the ocean. As they ascend from the cave, their leader becomes stuck in the entrance. The waters are rapidly rising and it is apparent that if the man is not freed from the entrance the others will drown. As it happens, a member of the group has some explosives. This gives the nine two choices. They can use the explosives on the person trapped in the entrance, thereby killing one but saving nine; or they can do nothing, thereby allowing one to live and nine to die. Now imagine someone using the doctrine of double effect and reasoning as follows:

> We are permitted to save the nine. The end of our act is to save nine people. The direct means to that end is to blow the man trapped in the entrance to bits. A foreseen but unintended consequence is that the man will be killed. But since the death of the man is neither the end sought nor the direct means to that end, we are permitted to bring about his death.

The criticism of this reasoning is not that it inappropriately permits the killing of one in order to save nine. This is a very difficult case and killing the trapped man may well be permitted. The criticism concerns the way in which the conclusion is derived. It seems to involve verbal manipulation. Describing the means to be employed as "blowing the man to bits" and the foreseen but unintended consequence as "the man will be killed" seems ludicrous. It is hard to imagine why it would be permissible to blow a person to bits but impermissible to kill that person. If a doctrine permits such sophistry, surely that is an argument against it. It seems that a sufficiently clever person could justify any conclusion through similar reasoning. Thus the doctrine of double effect should be rejected.

This criticism, however, may be unfair to advocates of the doctrine of double effect. It is clear that in the case presented the direct means and the foreseen but unintended consequence are two different descriptions of the same event. That is, "blowing the man to bits" and "the man's being killed" are two different ways of describing the same event. The defender of the doctrine of double effect can stipulate—and such a stipulaion would not be *ad hoc*—that a necessary condition for the correct application of this principle is that the means and the foreseen but unintended consequences described be two different events. Certainly in the emergency room case the event of devoting one-fifth of the physician's time and resources to each of five patients is distinct from the event of the sixth patient's dying. And the event of a woman carrying a child full term is distinct from, though causally related to, the woman's dying. This move at least provides defenders of the double effect doctrine with a response to this particular version of the verbal manipulation objection. However, this general sort of objection may still cause some difficulties. Suppose that the nine said that their end was to save their own lives and the means was to widen the entrance to the cave. Isn't widening the cave's entrance a different event from killing the man trapped there? And if so, doesn't this lend credence to the "verbal manipulation" objection? Moreover, even if the stipulation that the means and the foreseen but unintended consequence be different events does adequately answer the criticism, new questions are raised. How can a person tell when two different descriptions apply to the same event or when there are really two different events? And when there are a number of accurate descriptions of the same event, how does that person tell which is the morally relevant one? These are difficult questions that the advocate of the double effect principle must ponder.

In any case, there will be many who will reject the doctrine because of the particular moral judgments that it yields. Even though it does not fall prey to the problems of theses (I) and (II), they might argue, it still yields implausible moral judgments in certain cases. As already noted, some reject the doctrine of double effect because they believe that it forces its proponents to adopt the conservative position on the abortion issue. This, though, is not correct. This position on the abortion question follows only if additional assumptions about the nature of the fetus are made, assumptions that a defender of the doctrine of double effect need not make. There are, however, other moral judgments that the doctrine does yield which many find worrisome. Consider, for example, the case of a man trapped in a burning automobile. There is no way that you can save him, and realizing this, he pleads with you to shoot him (in order to spare him the pain of burning to death). The doctrine of double effect forbids such an act. The end of the act, of course, is to prevent suffering, but the direct means to that end involves killing the man. Thus, according to the doctrine, this may not be done. For this same reason, any act of mercy killing is forbidden. This, many contend, is too extreme. Thus there seem to be good reasons for doubting the adequacy of the doctrine of double effect.

## THE THEORY OF POSITIVE AND NEGATIVE DUTIES

Perhaps the best way to respond to the doctrine of double effect is to present an alternative theory. Philippa Foot has attempted this with her theory of positive and negative duties.[7] Let us begin by noting that many of the cases that theses (I) and (II) were designed to handle involved apparent conflicts of duties. This theory is designed to handle those conflicts. To begin, negative duties are duties to refrain from doing a certain thing. Typically, these are duties to avoid inflicting harm or injury on others. Thus the duties not to kill, not to steal, and not to torture others are negative duties. A positive duty is a duty to do a certain act, not merely refrain from doing something. Usually positive duties involve providing aid to or benefiting others. The duty to help an accident victim and the duty to save a drowning person are positive duties.

The theory of positive and negative duties is designed to handle conflict cases involving positive and negative duties. The theory consists of three clauses: (i) Whenever a negative duty conflicts with a positive duty, the negative duty always takes precedence. (ii) Whenever two negative duties conflict, an agent should do that act which brings about the lesser of the two evils. (iii) Whenever two positive duties conflict, an agent should do that act that brings about more good.

Let us explain clause (iii) first. The case of the six people brought to the emergency room involves a conflict of positive duties. On the one hand, there is a prima facie obligation to save the one person and this requires the physician to devote all available time and resources to that patient. On the other hand, there is a prima facie obligation to save the five patients and to do so the physician must devote an equal amount of time and resources to each of those patients. Clearly it is not possible to save the one patient and to save the other five patients. Since each of the duties in this conflict concerns bestowing benefits on others, clause (iii) directs the physician to choose the alternative that brings about more good. Thus the physician is required to save the five lives. It is regrettable that discharging this obligation will have as a consequence the death of the sixth patient. This strikes many people as the right thing to do in this case, and it is just the judgment that the theory of positive and negative duties yields.

Let us now consider clause (ii). No previous case seems to involve a conflict of negative duties, but the following does. Suppose that you find yourself at the controls of a runaway train. The braking mechanism on the train is inoperative. You are coming upon an intersection and can steer the train to the left or to the right. On the track to the left there are five people and on the track to the right there is one person. What should you do? All other things being equal, surely the thing to do in this tragic situation is to steer to the right. This involves the death of one person, but that alternative is preferable to killing five. This, of course, is precisely the judgment that clause (ii) yields. It tells us that when doing harm to others is inevitable, the lesser of two evils should be chosen.

According to clause (i), negative duties always override positive duties. To see how this works, let us reexamine the case of the five patients, each of whom needs an organ for transplantation in order to live. There is one available person who can serve as a suitable donor for each of the five, but obviously taking that person's vital organs will result in his or her death. There is a duty to do whatever can be done to save the five, but there is also a duty not to kill the one. The former of these duties is a positive one; the latter, negative. Clause (i) instructs us that the duty not to kill is the stronger and that therefore the five may not be saved at the expense of the one. And certainly that is the judgment that many people think is correct in this case.

If we confine ourselves only to these test cases, the theory of positive and negative duties yields plausible results. As might be expected, though, this theory has not gone uncriticized.[8] Perhaps the reader can construct cases in which this theory yields judgments that many people would find uncomfortable. To conclude, note that thesis (I), thesis (II), the doctrine of double effect, and the theory of positive and negative duties are alternative positions that yield different judgments on cases involving killing and letting die.

## EUTHANASIA:
## THE ISSUE AND SOME DISTINCTIONS

Euthanasia leads to moral problems because of the presence of conflicting values. Some values held by many tend to support the practice of euthanasia. First, it is believed in the abstract that people should have the right to make important choices that affect their own lives and harm no one else. This suggests that individuals who want to be mercy killed should be granted their wish. Second, most hold that it is morally desirable to prevent suffering. Since euthanasia sometimes advances this goal, that is another point in its favor. Finally, it is commonplace to say that "death with dignity" is a desirable end. Though it is not always clear what this means, it is usually thought that artificially prolonging the life of a person in an irreversible coma is a paradigmatic case of denying death with dignity. By contrast, however, there are some values that many hold that suggest euthanasia is wrong. Most people disapprove of intentionally taking the life of another human being. Since euthanasia normally involves doing just this, that counts against it. In addition, we are reluctant to institute a practice which can easily be abused and harm innocent persons. And, critics have argued, allowing people to be killed by their fellow human beings is a practice which it would be all too easy to abuse. There is a moral controversy about the practice of euthanasia, then, because it involves conflicting moral values.

Before discussing the question of when, if ever, euthanasia is permissible, some common distinctions must be explained. These distinctions have been thought by many to be morally relevant, and in any case they force us to focus more clearly on the issues involved. In examining these distinctions, it should be kept in mind that euthanasia is usually described as "mercy killing" or "easy death." This suggests that an act cannot accurately be described as one of euthanasia unless the motives or intentions of the actor are to do what is best for the person acted upon and the ensuing death is easy. The first distinction, then, is between active euthansia and passive euthansia. *Active euthanasia* is an action in which the death of a person is induced by doing something to end his or her life when it would otherwise go on. Thus the agent of the person's death is actively interfering in the course of natural events. Active euthanasia is a form of killing (as opposed to letting die). *Passive euthanasia* is allowing death to come more quickly by terminating extraordinary treatment or refraining from initiating such treatment. A person who engages in passive euthanasia is simply letting nature take its course; the person is letting the other die (as opposed to killing the other). Injecting a suffering person with a lethal drug would be a case of active euthanasia. Disconnecting a person in an irreversible coma from a respirator or failing to connect the person in the first place is usually described as a case of passive euthanasia. The qualification "extraordinary" is included because most do not want to say that allowing a person to die from starvation is a case of passive euthanasia (though, as will be seen, there are exceptions). It must be admitted, however, that the distinction between extraordinary and ordinary treatment is difficult to draw.

The second distinction is between voluntary and involuntary euthanasia. *Voluntary euthanasia* is killing the patient or letting the patient die only when he or she consents to or requests that this be done. *Involuntary euthanasia* is killing the patient or letting the patient die when he or she has neither consented to nor requested that this be done. When engaging in voluntary euthanasia, a person is simply abiding by the expressed wishes of that person whose death is induced. When engaging in involuntary euthanasia, a person is deciding for another person that death is preferable to living, given the conditions under which that person must live. Involuntary euthanasia is deciding for another what is best for him or her.

The differences to which these distinctions call attention are thought by many to be morally relevant. How this is so can be explained in the following way. On the basis of these two distinctions, four different cases can be differentiated: (i) involuntary active euthanasia; (ii) involuntary passive euthanasia; (iii) voluntary active euthanasia; and (iv) voluntary passive euthanasia. Arranging the possible cases in this way, some have claimed, enables us to rate them in terms of the degrees of their moral seriousness. Thus a fairly standard way of arguing is this: involuntary euthanasia is always more serious than voluntary euthanasia and active euthanasia is always more serious than passive euthanasia. To say that one act is more serious than another is simply to say that it is more difficult to justify morally. It might be held, then, that case (i) is the case of euthanasia most difficult to justify and that case (iv) is the least difficult to justify. Ordering cases (ii) and (iii) is apt to produce more disagreement, but a not uncommon position is that (ii) is more serious than (iii). It is important to realize that advocates of two very extreme positions—that no form of euthanasia is ever permissible and that any form of euthanasia may be permissible—might agree about arranging cases (i) through (iv). That is, a person who thinks that euthanasia is always wrong might still agree that it would be easier to justify voluntary passive euthanasia than it would be to justify involuntary active euthanasia. Similarly, a person who believes that any form of euthanasia may be justified might agree that it is more difficult to justify cases of type (i) than it is to justify any of the other types of cases.

Few will disagree that there is a morally relevant difference between voluntary and involuntary euthanasia. Even those who hold that all forms of euthanasia are impermissible acknowledge that involuntary euthanasia is more serious than voluntary euthanasia. There is less harmony, however, concerning the alleged difference between active euthanasia and passive euthanasia. Within the medical and legal communities, though, there does seem to be considerable agreement that this distinction is morally important. Consider the following statement issued by the American Medical Association in December, 1973.[9]

> The intentional termination of the life of one human being by another—mercy killing—is contrary to that for which the medical profession stands and is contrary to the policy of the American Medical Association.
>
> The cessation of the employment of extraordinary means to prolong the life of the body when there is irrefutable evidence that biological death is imminent is the decision of the patient and/or his immediate family. The advice and judgment of the physician should be freely available to the patient and/or his immediate family.

A careful analysis of this statement shows that the AMA endorses two claims: (1) There is a morally relevant difference between active euthanasia and passive euthanasia and (2) the difference is such that active euthanasia is never permissible but voluntary passive euthanasia is permissible if the death of the patient is imminent. The AMA, then, is committed to the claim that passive euthanasia is less serious, from the moral point of view, than active euthanasia. Passive euthanasia is permitted, though, only if it is voluntary. They do extend the notion of "voluntary," however, to cover cases where members of the immediate family consent for the patient. Though they do not say this, it is presumed that such proxy consent will occur only when the patient is unable to speak for himself or herself, such as when the patient is unconscious.

A similar position has been taken by some members of the legal community. To illustrate this, a brief discussion of the famous case of Karen Quinlan will follow. The facts of this case are well known. Karen was a twenty-one year old who was comatose. Physicians agreed that her state was irreversible, that she would never regain consciousness. Her vital life processes were being sustained artificially by a respirator. Karen's parents requested that the respirator be disconnected. The hospital refused to go along with their wishes, and eventually the case went to court. Initially the decision went against the Quinlans. In November, 1975, Judge Robert Muir, Jr., of the Superior Court of New Jersey refused to grant the request of the Quinlans that the respirator be disconnected. Later, however, in a decision written by Justice C.J. Hughes, the Supreme Court of New Jersey reversed this decision.[10] The respirator was turned off, though at the time of this writing Karen Quinlan is alive but comatose.

For our purposes, there are three important points made in the opinion of Justice Hughes. (i) It was claimed that the (presumed) ensuing death of Karen Quinlan would not be homicide. Rather it would be "expiration from natural causes." There is a legally important difference, it was argued, between the unlawful taking of the life of another and the ending of artificial life-support systems upon request. In short, they suggest that there is a relevant difference between killing and letting die, and by implication they indicate that only the latter might be permitted in cases of this sort. (ii) The court argued that the focal point of the decision in cases like this should be on the prognosis. In particular, the crucial issue is whether there is a reasonable possibility of return to cognitive life as distinguished from forced continuance of mere biological existence. And in Karen's case there was no reasonable chance of return to cognitive life. (iii) Not only did members of the immediate family request that the respirator be disconnected, but there was also some evidence that Karen herself would not have wanted her life sustained artificially in such circumstances. The testamonies of a friend and a family member indicated that Karen had stated that she would not want to be kept alive artificially if there were no hope for her recovery. It can be seen, then, that the decision of the Supreme Court of New Jersey is very much in accord with the statement issued by the AMA. The decision suggests that removing Karen from the respirator is permissible only because it is a case of voluntary passive euthanasia.

## LEGALIZING EUTHANASIA

There is much debate today concerning legalizing euthanasia. Many different pieces of euthanasia legislation have been proposed. Here we shall indicate the sort of questions that must be asked in assessing any proposal. A discussion of several objections that have been raised against legalizing euthanasia will also ensue. These objections are, in effect, moral criticisms of some of the various proposals. In coming to grips with any proposed piece of legislation concerning euthanasia, it is useful to raise four questions. (1) Who are the possible subjects or the candidates for euthanasia? That is, if this legislative proposal were adopted, whom would it be permissible to mercy kill? (2) Does the proposal allow for only voluntary euthanasia, or does it allow for involuntary euthanasia too? (3) Does the proposal allow for both passive and active euthanasia, or does it allow for just one of these? (4) What safeguards are built into the legislation in order to protect against the possibility of abuse? Each of these questions will be considered.

Let us turn first to question (1). Obviously different legislative proposals include different groups as the possible subjects of euthanasia. However, the following four categories are those most often included. First, persons who have painful and terminal diseases such as throat cancer are thought to be plausible candidates. These are people who will die soon anyway and who will be in excruciating pain until death occurs. It is often said that denying them the right to be mercy killed upon request is to force them to suffer for no reason. Thus this group is frequently included in legislation to support euthanasia because it is desirable to minimize human suffering. Second, many argue that euthanasia should be an option for those who are permanently unconscious. Persons who are in an irreversible coma are often called "human vegetables." Though their continued existence is not painful, it is claimed that it is meaningless. Often people in this state are being kept alive by artificial means (for example, by being connected to a respirator). Sometimes, however, they remain alive if only ordinary treatment is continued (for example, intravenous feeding)—note the case of Karen Quinlan. The rationale for including persons in this category is, it is said, to promote "death with dignity." Third, it is sometimes suggested that severely deformed infants are beings on whom it should be permissible to practice euthanasia. These are infants who suffer from gross mental or physical defects. In some cases the life expectancy of children in this group is very short; in other cases their life expectancy is fairly normal. In either case, though, the life that the child will live will be very unsatisfying. Finally, it is sometimes suggested that severely retarded adults or persons suffering from senility are persons on whom mercy killing may be practiced. The recent case of a seventy-eight year old Massachusetts man, Earle Spring, falls under this last category. Mr. Spring had been declared incompetent—he was apparently severely senile. For more than two years he had had to spend five hours on a kidney dialysis machine three times a week. Without such treatment, Earle Spring would die. In January of 1979 Spring's family requested that the treatment be stopped. Since Spring was suffering no pain, it would seem that their reason for making this request was directly connected with his senility. Initially, the courts ruled in the family's favor. However, a nurse and a doctor claimed that Mr. Spring had expressed a desire to live, and so the treatments were resumed.

Question (2) may be answered by saying that usually a proposed piece of legislation advocates only voluntary euthanasia; allowing for involuntary euthanasia seems to many to go too far.[11] There is some question, though, about what cases may be included under the description "voluntary euthanasia." Usually it is said that euthanasia is voluntary if consent is obtained. But exactly what form must this consent take? There are at least three possibilities here. A very narrow notion of voluntary euthanasia, holding that a person has consented only if he or she has specifically requested, here and now, that the act take place, might be adopted. This conception is narrow because unless a person is able to (and does) make his or her request known at the time the act is desired, no consent has been given. A second notion of voluntary euthanasia is more liberal in that it allows for a person to consent by stating his or her wishes in advance. The person may specify that if certain conditions obtain, he or she does not wish to be kept alive. Documents that have come to be known as "living wills" enable a person to convey his or her wishes in this way. There is still a more liberal notion of voluntary euthanasia that includes not only the patient's consent, but also allows for proxy consent. Proxy consent is when one person consents on behalf of another. Thus a parent, a child, a spouse or a sibling may consent to euthanasia for you. Of course, proxy consent cannot in any literal sense be a person's own voluntary act. But if it is assumed, not unreasonably, that a parent, child, spouse, or sibling knows what the patient's wishes would be and acts to see that those are fulfilled, then there is some sense in which what the patient wants is being taken into account.

It is important to realize that how the notion of consent is interpreted is not merely an abstract, verbal dispute. For obvious reasons, few are willing to advocate involuntary euthanasia. But if the cases of legally permitted mercy killings are limited to those involving consent, then absolute clarity on what counts as consent must be sought. And notice the practical implications. Suppose the narrow interpretation of consent is adopted: euthanasia is voluntary only if the patient has directly consented, here and now. Of the four groups or types of cases where mercy killing might be desirable, only the first—persons who are suffering from a painful, terminal illness—is one in which the patient can directly consent. Clearly unconscious persons, infants, and senile persons are not capable of giving direct consent. If the notion of voluntary euthanasia is extended to include expressing individual wishes in advance, then this will allow for the possibility of euthanasia for those who are permanently unconscious or severely senile. It will be permissible to engage in euthanasia in these two types of cases, however, only if the persons in question have explicitly communicated in advance their wishes that this be done. Those who have remained silent about such matters will, on this view, have to be kept alive. Clearly, though, infants are not capable of giving any sort of consent. Thus if euthanasia is restricted to voluntary euthanasia and if euthanasia for severely deformed infants is desirable, then proxy consent will have to be allowed. Whether it is desirable to open the door this widely, however, is a question that must be asked.

Question (3) asks whether a proposed statute allows for only passive euthanasia, active euthanasia, or both. As previously seen, in both the medical and legal communities there seems to be a deeply entrenched belief that passive euthanasia is more acceptable than active euthanasia. In fact, active euthanasia is identified with killing and is said always to be wrong. Notice, though, the consequences of limiting legally permitted acts of euthanasia to the passive cases only. Many cases where people believe that euthanasia is desirable will be cases where it is forbidden: for example, the case of the person suffering from a painful, terminal illness. If euthanasia is desirable here, its purpose is to relieve needless suffering. But this purpose can be achieved only if active euthanasia is performed. Obviously the person in this case is going to die soon anyway. The point is to relieve the person of suffering and passive euthanasia cannot accomplish this. Passive euthanasia will achieve its purpose in only some of the other three types of cases. Certainly some people who are permanently unconscious will die if extraordinary means of life support, such as a respirator, are discontinued. But certainly not all will; Karen Quinlan serves as a vivid reminder of that. If the goal of euthanasia in these cases is to end a meaningless existence or allow a person to die with dignity, passive euthansia will achieve this only in some of the cases. The same is true of persons in the last two categories: severly deformed infants and the very senile. Sometimes these people are being kept alive by extraordinary medical treatment; but sometimes only the most mundane sort of treatment is needed. Thus allowing for only passive euthanasia will be thought as too restrictive by many.

One other point is worth noting concerning the difference between active and passive euthanasia. Despite the strong bias to the contrary, in some cases it seems obvious that passive euthanasia is worse, from the moral point of view, than active euthanasia. Cases have been reported where physicians (and perhaps the parents) have judged that infant euthanasia is desirable because of the severe deformities of the child. The physician, being opposed to active euthanasia, then orders the attending nurses to quit feeding the child, and to let it die of starvation. Euthanasia, though, is supposed to be an act of mercy. How anyone can think that starving an infant to death is more merciful than killing it painlessly and quickly is a great mystery. If any form of infant euthanasia is permissible in a case like this, surely it is only active euthanasia.

Question (4) asks what safeguards are built into the legislation to protect against the possibility of abuse. The worry, of course, is that if one human being is allowed to take the life of another, things may get out of hand. Many safeguards have been proposed by those who favor enacting euthanasia legislation, but only a few will be mentioned here. One safeguard usually suggested is to restrict euthanasia to those who have themselves requested the act. A second is to require that the patient be a legal adult, say eighteen years old. This presumably is designed to prevent those who are too immature from making such an irreversible decision. Third, many specify that the agent of the act (that is, the person who does the mercy killing) must be a physician who has consulted with at least one other physician. The requirement of consultation is designed to minimize medical errors. Before engaging in euthanasia, physicians must be as sure as they can that the case is hopeless. The requirement that the agent be a physician is apparently paternalistic, and perhaps justifiable. If anyone were permitted to engage in euthanasia, a patient temporarily in great pain may ask someone with no medical knowledge to aid him or her in hastening his or her death. A qualified medical person may refuse, however, because he or she knows that this painful condition is only temporary. The person's request is irrational because he or she will be able to return to normalcy; but only someone with expertise in medical matters would know this. Finally, some suggest that a certain period of time must elapse between the time of the request and the act itself. This, of course, is designed to ensure that the person really wants to die; it allows for changes of mind at the last minute. Again, this safeguard is justified, if at all, on paternalistic grounds.

There is, of course, a great controversy concerning the question of legalizing euthanasia. What sort of reasons have been given to defend the claim that euthanasia should be legally permissible? Proponents have contended that voluntary euthanasia promotes and upholds two widely shared values. First, few, if any, would disagree that it is desirable to prevent cruelty and needless suffering. A person who is in great pain, is terminally ill, and requests that death be hastened, is suffering needlessly and for no purpose. In a case like this not only does euthanasia prevent suffering for the subject, but it also relieves the agony of the relatives who must watch the subject's slow and painful death. Liberty or personal autonomy is the second value that voluntary euthanasia promotes. Many argue that the criminal law should be invoked to repress conduct only if doing so prevents harm to others (in particular, nonconsenting adults or children). Forbidding voluntary euthanasia is not necessary to prevent harm to others. So, the argument concludes, it should not be prohibited.

Not everyone will find these reasons persuasive. The usual objection to legalizing invountary euthanasia is to claim that such an act is murder (at least if it is active euthanasia). Involuntary euthanasia deprives a person of his or her right to life. Moreover, it is a violation of a person's autonomy. Perhaps a person may waive his or her own right to life. Others, however, may not make such a decision. Certainly members of the health care team do not have such an option. Some may want to extend this argument further and claim that a spouse, child, sibling, or parent may not give others permission to end another's life either. On this view, proxy consent is not allowed and euthanasia in such a case is involuntary. It is important to note that if this account of involuntary euthanasia is accepted and if no case of involuntary euthanasia is permissible, then it follows that infant euthanasia is absolutely forbidden.

Why, though, have people objected to allowing for voluntary euthanasia? Why is it wrong for a society to allow its citizens to choose death for themselves in these extreme cases? Many objections have been raised to legalizing even voluntary euthanasia, and some of these will be articulated here.

First, even if the victim consents and the actor's motives (i.e., the agent of death) are humanitarian, the critic contends that this provides no legal or moral defense for killing. Certainly most people agree that if a person walks up to you on the street and asks you to kill him or her, you are not justified in doing so. The same is true, it is argued, in the case of voluntary euthanasia. This objection seems to rest on the claim that the right to life is inalienable. A right is inalienable just in case it may not be waived or transferred by its possessor. A right is alienable if it may be waived or transferred by its possessor. To say that some rights are alienable is uncontroversial. Certainly property rights are alienable. Since you purchased this book, you have property rights to it. You may give this book to a friend; in so doing, you have transferred the property rights to him or her. You have property rights to the land that you purchased. You may, however, waive some of those rights and allow me to walk across it daily in order to arrive at my destination more quickly. Some rights are not like this, though, according to the critic. The rights to life, liberty, and the pursuit of happiness are inalienable according to Thomas Jefferson. Thus even voluntary euthanasia is impermissible.

The second objection to legalizing voluntary euthanasia is presented in the form of a dilemma. It concerns the desirability of including safeguards in any statute permitting euthanasia. If all of the necessary restrictions are included in the legislation, it is claimed, very few people will benefit and the main purposes of euthanasia will have been lost. The following are some of the points the critic makes to establish this horn of the dilemma: if we permit only voluntary euthanasia, then many persons who are permanently unconscious will not qualify under the act; if only passive euthanasia is permitted, then we will be unable to prevent the needless suffering of those with a painful, terminal illness; and if a time lapse is required between the request and the act, additional needless suffering will occur. On the other hand, if the necessary safeguards are not included in the law, then the possibility of abuse (by relatives, physicians, and others) is much too great. The conditions under which one human being is allowed to end the life of another must be carefully restricted. Thus proponents of legalizing euthanasia face a difficult dilemma.

A third objection appeals to alleged medical facts. It is claimed that the humanitarian goal of preventing suffering can be achieved without ending the patient's life. The many modern techniques for controlling pain, including tranquilizers, narcotics, and anesthetics should be used to keep the patient alive and painless as long as possible.

It is often difficult to tell when a person has genuinely consented to the act of mercy killing. This provides the basis for the fourth objection: what appears to be a case of voluntary euthanasia may not be one at all. To support this criticism, the following claims are made. If consent is given in the final stages of a painful illness, during moments of great pain or under the influence of heavy sedation, there will be doubts about the rationality of the patient and hence about his or her capability of giving consent. Of course, the person may have given consent in advance, either by signing a "living will" or by communicating his or her wishes verbally. But even in this sort of case doubts can arise. And there is the possibility that the person has changed his or her mind. In the case of a living will, it is reasonable to expect that if the person did undergo a change of mind, the person would disavow the document and have it destroyed. When the wishes have been communicated verbally, however, this is much less likely. In fact, whether the person was even serious when these desires were expressed may be difficult to determine. Karen Quinlan, when normal, supposedly expressed to others the wish not to be kept alive artificially if there was no hope for recovery. But was she serious when she said this? Had she given the matter much thought? And isn't there the possibility that she subsequently changed her mind? There is another problem with consent given in advance. A person may specify that he or she does not want to be kept alive if certain conditions obtain. It may be difficult to determine, though, whether these conditions do in fact obtain. The source of the difficulty is twofold. First, the conditions may have been vaguely specified by the person. Second, the person may have stated that he or she did not want to be kept alive if he or she were terminally ill. Doubts will occasionally arise here because there will be some uncertainty as to whether the condition is in fact terminal. The first of these two sources of doubt is more serious. A final point concerning the difficulty of determining whether consent is genuine appeals to the possibility that others may want the patient to consent. The patient may feel some pressure to consent to death in order to relieve the relatives or family members of their suffering.

A fifth objection to legalizing voluntary euthanasia appeals to the nature of the decision. The choice to have one's life ended is irrevocable. In general, it is claimed, a person should avoid making irrevocable decisions whenever possible. It is a canon of rationality that a person should keep as many options open to himself or herself as possible. And in a decision involving euthanasia, the stakes are very high. The consequences of making a foolish, irrevocable decision in such cases are fatal. Thus there should not be laws permitting people to make such choices.

The sixth objection, closely related to the fifth, asserts that the judgment that a person is terminally ill may be mistaken in two ways.

First, there is always the possibility of a simple diagnostic error. The physician may judge that the patient has a certain terminal illness, when in fact the patient has a different disease, which is curable. If the physician consults with another doctor, the possibility of such an error is lessened; but it is still a possibility. Second, a new cure may be found for the illness after the patient has been mercy killed but before he or she would have died of natural causes. Thus, contrary to the physician's belief, the patient could have been saved.

The wedge argument is the final objection to legalizing voluntary euthanasia that will be considered here. According to this criticism, voluntary euthanasia ought not be legalized because the consequences of doing so will be disastrous. Advocates of the wedge argument claim that if voluntary euthanasia is permitted, other sorts of euthanasia will (inevitably?) follow. If voluntary euthanasia is legalized, these critics maintain, a relaxation in the present strong prohibition against killing will result. And once the absolute value placed on human life is diminished, the concept of voluntary euthanasia will be stretched to cover more and more cases. Ultimately, approval of involuntary euthanasia will result. This in turn will lead our society to approve of euthanasia for the so-called social undesirables, namely, the severely retarded and the senile. Finally, the door may be opened wide enough so that a despot can use the euthanasia legislation to justify activities of the sort that Hitler engaged in, cases in which people are exterminated because of their race or ethnic background. Since these consequences are clearly undesirable, they must be prevented. And this can be done, the critic argues, only if euthanasia is stopped at the outset. Specific evidence is rarely produced to support these claims, but this is an often cited objection to legalizing euthanasia.

Proponents of legalizing voluntary euthanasia have not been convinced by these objections. To deal with their replies in detail, however, would require a lengthy discussion. A brief and superficial indication of how the proponent might respond to these objections will be given. The reader will be able to develop the suggestions further as he or she sees fit.

To the first objection that a person may not consent to his or her own death, the proponent usually denies the assumption upon which this is predicated. The person argues that the right to life is not inalienable; in any case, voluntary euthanasia is not a typical situation of consenting to death because the subject usually will die soon anyway, or at least be permanently comatose.[12] To the second criticism, the dilemma, the defender of euthanasia responds that even if it is true that only a few will benefit when the necessary safeguards are included, that is no reason to delay the legislation. If even a few can benefit surely they should be allowed to do so. Moreover, the proponent has serious doubts that only a few will be beneficiaries of such legislation. According to the third objection the goal of preventing suffering can be achieved through the use of pain-killing drugs and so euthanasia need not be engaged in. Those who favor voluntary euthanasia say that this is true only in some cases. In other cases, however, the pain and suffering can be stopped only if the patient is killed. Sometimes the suffering can be prevented only if the dosage of the pain-killing drug is so strong that the medical worker knows it will directly induce death. The death of the patient may not be the intended end of the medical worker's act, but to say that this is not a case of mercy killing is incredible.

The fourth objection is designed to make us skeptical about our ability to know when consent is genuine or really voluntary. In general, the advocate of voluntary euthanasia says that this criticism is based on a series of exaggerated claims. Of course, there are some cases where it is difficult for us to tell if the consent is genuine, but on the whole this is a matter about which such extreme skepticism is out of place. The response to the fifth objection is that not all irrevocable decisions are irrational. That a certain decision will be irrevocable is not a reason for not making it at all; it is simply a reason for being very cautious before one makes it. The sixth objection can be defused, it is argued, for the following reasons. It is true, of course, that the physician may make a diagnostic error. But if he or she consults with another physician, these will be minimized. And in any case, even if an occasional error is tragically made, the issue is the overall balance of pain and pleasure. Should many people be denied relief from suffering simply because if they are allowed this relief there will be rare cases that result in the deaths of persons who could have been saved? To the second part of this objection, the defender of euthanasia charges that the critic is operating with an extremely naive and unrealistic picture of medical discovery. The critic seems to think that a scientific breakthrough made today will result in the mass production of the miracle cure tomorrow. But this is not the way discovery in medical contexts works. After the initial breakthrough, much testing is required before the drug may be used on human beings. Several years may elapse between the time of the breakthrough and the general availability of the cure. And, assuming that the physician keeps up with the current research in his or her field, then the physician will know whether the initial breakthrough has been made and will so inform the patient. Finally, the response to the seventh objection, the wedge argument, is simple. What is the evidence to support these claims? To assert that a causal consequence of legalizing voluntary euthanasia will be the mercy killing of the retarded and the senile is a claim that requires justification. Unless evidence is produced to support this claim, there is no reason to believe it. It sometimes seems that the wedge argument involves an appeal to scare tactics, but of course its proponents contend that there are good reasons to be frightened.[13]

These, then, are the basic issues concerning the question of legalizing voluntary euthanasia. Although no arguments for any final conclusions concerning this topic have been presented, a framework has been provided in which the reader can place and argue for his or her own views.

## INFANT EUTHANASIA

The issue of infant euthanasia is treated as a separate topic because there is no possibility of the subject consenting in these cases: the parents or medical workers must make the final decision. Whether infant euthanasia can ever be voluntary depends on how loosely one uses the term "voluntary." If the notion of voluntary euthanasia is stretched to include proxy consent, then infant euthanasia can be voluntary. If, however, the notion is restricted to apply only to cases where the subject has directly or indirectly consented, then infant euthanasia can never be voluntary. It is doubtful that much hangs on this verbal dispute. In the case where infant euthansia is passive and requested by the parents, we have a special case of a legal guardian refusing lifesaving therapy for a dependent. It is a special case because to describe it as euthanasia suggests that the principal motive of the guardian is the well-being of the infant. Active infant euthanasia, however, goes byond the refusal of lifesaving therapy; it involves hastening the infant's death through some positive act.

There are two types of cases where some are inclined to advocate infant euthanasia. The first type of case is that in which there is overwhelming evidence that the child will die relatively soon anyway, no matter what is done. This death can be prolonged, however, if certain treatment is initiated. The treatment that will extend the life of the child may be extraordinary, such as the use of a respirator, or it may be less exotic, such as the performance of routine surgery. In either case, though, the options are two: if nothing is done, the child will die immediately; if the treatment is initiated, it is believed that the child will live longer but will still die in a relatively short period of time.

In the second type of case, the infant can be saved but at a great expense. In this type of case, if nothing is done, the infant probably will die soon. But if treatment is initiated, the infant will be able to live more or less indefinitely. The expense incurred is the great burden that must be borne if the infant is saved. Financial and emotional burdens will fall on the parents. There may also be burdens on the infant itself. If the baby's condition is severe and painful enough, it may be plausible to say that merely existing is burdensome. Great care must be exercised in saying that life itself may be burdensome. It might be suggested, though, that such a claim is reasonable in the case of babies with myelomeningocele, a particularly tragic form of spina bifida with a portion of cord and membranes protruding. (Spina bifida is a congenital defect in the walls of the spinal canal caused by a lack of union between the laminaie of the vertebrae. Because of the spinal cord deformity, the victim is paralyzed below the level of the injury.) But it is not plausible to say this in the case of a baby with Down's syndrome (also called mongolism), since the evidence suggests that such children can live relatively contented lives, although the quality of those lives may be judged low by others' standards.

It appears to be easier to justify infant euthanasia in the first type of case, where a parent or guardian can appeal to the interests of the infant itself. Prolonging the child's death, it might be argued, is of no benefit even to the child. In this situation there is nothing to be gained by initiating treatment. By contrast, in the second type of case the interests of others are often invoked in an attempt to justify infant euthanasia. Now in some cases a parent or guardian might also appeal to the interests of the infant itself; the extreme case of spina bifida provides an example here. But in other cases, an appeal to the interests of the infant itself will not be plausible, such as in the case of a Mongoloid child. Not infrequently Mongoloid children will have an additional medical problem, such as a heart defect, which can be corrected with simple surgery. Parents of these children are sometimes tempted to refuse to give permission for the surgery, thus letting the infant die. It cannot plausibly be claimed, however, that this is done for the interests of the child itself. The evidence suggests that Mongoloid children live contented but simple lives. If infant euthansia were ever justified in the case of Mongoloid children, it would have to involve an appeal to the interests of others.

Is it ever appropriate to justify infant euthanasia by appealing to the interests of others? Although there will be no attempt to settle this question here, it is worth noting that in certain extreme cases the claim that it is justified does not seem to be completely implausible. Robert Veatch presents a case that may lead one to entertain seriously the idea that one may appeal to the interests of others.[14] This case involves a baby who had an open myelomeningocele. With surgery, there was a 70 to 75 percent chance that the child would live. But there was a good chance that if the child survived it would be unable to walk without the aid of braces, its intelligence would be adversely affected, and the cost for caring for the child in terms of time and money would be very great. As it happened, the parents of this child were not wealthy and had three other children. Moreover, there was evidence that their oldest child was having difficulty in school and would require special attention. These parents considered refusing to give permission for the surgery not because they did not want such a child but because of the likely consequences on their other three children. Because of their very limited income, they were afraid that they would be unable to care adequately for their other children. In this case appealing to the interests of others to justify infant euthansia does not seem as callous as it does when the parents simply do not want to have a Mongoloid child. Whether this is a legitimate case of infant euthanasia, however, is a matter for further debate. Presumably, though, most people prefer to see a policy adopted which does not kill a deformed infant simply because the family cannot afford to care for it. This is surely a case where it is legitimate for the state to offer assistance in funding the medical bills of some of its citizens.

Some birth defects are severe. The prospects for a child born with spina bifida are not good, and other birth defects are even worse. These are cases where a parent or guardian might be able to appeal plausibly to the interests of the infant itself to justify euthanasia. What should be done in such a case? There are at least three responses that can be made. (i) Everything within our power to save these children should be done, no matter what the cost is (to the child itself or to others). Those who favor this view say that the purpose of medicine is to save lives and someone should never be allowed to die who can be saved. (ii) At the other extreme, some advocate killing these babies. The suffering that they must endure is too great and there is no reasonable chance that they will recover. In addition, the financial and emotional burden on their parents is too great. It is an act of mercy to end the suffering of these children quickly. (iii) These children should not be actively killed, but positive steps to keep them alive should not be taken either. The appropriate policy is to let them die. This is thought to be a compromise between the first two positions. It seems to be the predominant view in the medical community and is expressed in different ways. Some suggest that it is appropriate to "let Nature take its course."[15] Or, as others say, "Nature if left alone will always correct its own mistakes in these cases."[16]

Position (i) advocates the heroic line of saving every infant possible; position (ii) defends active infant euthanasia; position (iii) supports passive infant euthanasia. These three positions, it would seem, exhaust the alternatives. Yet each seems unsatisfactory. Position (i) seems to place too great an emotional and financial burden on the parents and family members of the infant. In some cases the sacrifice is so great that it might be said that if the family chooses to make it they have engaged in a supererogatory act; in any case, they are not required to bear such a burden. Second, if the birth defects are severe (as is supposed), it is not clear that it is in the interests of the child to save it. As one author puts it, "Will they [the seriously deformed children] really be grateful to the fates, the all too human fates, but for whose intervention they would have died before their miseries began?"[17] Third, it may not be in society's interest to save these infants. There is a good chance that many of these children who survive will have to be kept or aided by society. And if by chance any of them should have children of their own, there may be a danger that the defect in question will be passed on to future generations.

There are also objections to position (ii). This position advocates directly killing the infants. But to many this seems too extreme. It is inappropriate, they argue, for medical workers, whose chief purpose it is to save lives, to engage in activities that end lives. Moreover, the victim in these cases is someone who cannot consent. Finally, if the reason that infant euthanasia is desirable is that the child will be a burden to others, the wedge argument may be invoked against this practice. After all, those who are not deformed may also be a burden to their parents and so to allow this may open the door to infanticide in general. Is an ugly child too much of a burden to its parents? Is a child of the unpreferred sex too much of a burden?

Because of these difficulties many have opted for position (iii). As suggested earlier, this does seem to be the predominant view among members of the medical community. Its appeal is that it does not saddle parents with a great burden, nor does it require medical workers to kill the child. However, it can be argued that this is the least acceptable of the three positions. What this position overlooks (or ignores) is that many infants with these defects do not die soon. Some live for months, dying slow, agonizing deaths. Others live for years. Often the attempt to let these children die involves refusing surgery for some other, easily correctable medical problem. When these infants do not die soon, their problems have been compounded. That is, if they survive in spite of the fact that they have been denied ordinary treatment that any other child would have received, the quality of their lives is even worse than it would have been had they received optimal treatment. Given these facts, it is hard to see why so many favor the policy of letting die. The degree to which the policy of letting die is favored over the other two cannot be exaggerated. As was mentioned earlier, it has been reported that some physicians have ordered nurses to quit feeding a severely deformed infant. This, of course, will insure that the child will die. But why would anyone think that this is preferable to directly killing the infant? Letting die in this way is most assuredly not merciful. If for whatever reasons it has been decided (by the medical team and the parents) that it would be better if the infant were to die, surely killing it quickly and painlessly is far better than starving it to death. To hold that letting die is always better than killing, even when it requires starvation, is moral lunacy.

If this argument is correct, position (iii), in spite of its popularity, is the least acceptable policy to adopt regarding severely deformed infants. But which of the other two is preferable? One possibility is that either of the first two alternatives be left open to parents of these children. Some may opt for active euthanasia; some may prefer to do everything possible to save the child. Certainly if the parents want to save the child and are willing to bear the costs of doing so, society should not prevent this. And, of course, there is no reason to believe that just one of these policies must be adopted; perhaps different situations call for different responses. At this point, though, it will be left to the reader to wrestle with the pros and the cons of positions (i) and (ii).[18]

## ADULT EUTHANASIA

Why is adult euthanasia a separate topic from infant euthanasia? Adults, unlike infants, are capable of consenting to their own death. With adults, voluntary euthanasia is a possibility. It is sometimes said that voluntary euthanasia is no different than suicide. The two do, of course, have one obvious thing in common: each is an instance of a person wishing for and seeking death. There does seem to be an important difference, however. Suicide involves only one party, namely, the person who wants to die; voluntary euthanasia, however, involves a second party, the person aiding the one who wants to die. And this may be a morally relevant difference since allowing a second party to be the instrument of a person's death opens the door to possible abuses of the sort to which the wedge argument calls attention. This suggests that some will want to deny the claim that if suicide is sometimes permissible, then voluntary euthanasia will be permissible too.

To deny the converse, however, is less plausible. It seems quite reasonable to say that if suicide is always wrong, then voluntary euthanasia is also always wrong. Put another way, suicide is no more morally problematic than voluntary euthanasia and it may well be less problematic. Suppose that suicide were always wrong. What could possibly allow someone else to end your life at your request when you yourself are not permitted to take such an action? If this is correct, it lays the groundwork for an objection to voluntary adult euthanasia that must be considered. Opponents may argue that voluntary adult euthanasia is impermissible because suicide is always wrong. If these opponents can convince us that suicide is always wrong, this will be a very forceful objection. In order to deal with this objection, proponents of euthanasia will need to do two things. First, they will need to consider the reasons the critic gives to show that suicide is always wrong and demonstrate that those reasons are inadequate. Second, they will need to present a positive case to convince us that suicide is at least sometimes permissible.

Why, then, have some thought that suicide is always wrong? Of course, a number of different reasons have been given by those who believe that suicide is always wrong. Many of these reasons are religious in nature and they will not be considered here. Instead our focus will consider two secular arguments designed to show that suicide is impermissible. The first is called the natural law argument. According to this argument, suicide is wrong because it is unnatural. Suicide involves a breach of the natural law of self-preservation. It is assumed, of course, that doing what is unnatural is wrong. This sort of argument is not atypical. Many argue that homosexuality and other forms of so-called deviant sexual behavior are immoral because they are unnatural. Indeed, a view often associated with St. Thomas Aquinas is that any form of sexual activity not aimed at reproduction is unnatural and therefore wrong. To say that self-preservation is a natural law is to say that each living creature is endowed with the instinct for self-preservation. Yet it is difficult to understand this argument. It appears to derive what a person ought to do from premises that state what is the case. Some would say that this alone shows that the argument fails because it commits what philosophers call the naturalistic fallacy.[19]

A different tack can be taken in criticizing the argument, however. In what sense is the law of self-preservation a law? There are at least two senses of "law" that might be meant here, but investigation will show that on either account the argument is inadequate. The term "natural law" might be used in the descriptive sense. This means that the law describes how things are. Such laws are universal in scope. Thus Newton's laws of gravity are natural laws in the descriptive sense. If the claim that the law of self-preservation is a law in the descriptive sense, then clearly it is false. Not every being seeks to preserve itself; clearly those who commit suicde show that it is not a natural law in the descriptive sense. The term "natural law" might also be used in the prescriptive sense, though. This means that the law tells us not how things are but rather how they ought to be. The law prohibiting the killing of innocent persons is a prescriptive law. Perhaps the advocate of the natural law argument intends the law of self-preservation to be understood as a prescriptive law. If so, the argument will not be subject to the simple counterexample presented above. However, it will be open to another serious objection. If the law of self-preservation is taken to be a prescriptive law, the argument will be question-begging. To say that an argument is question-begging is to say that it presupposes the truth of the proposition to be proved. If the law of self-preservation is understood to be a prescriptive law, then presumably it tells us that there is an obligation to preserve oneself. But to say that an individual ought to preserve his or her life is just to say that attempting suicide is wrong, and so the truth of the conclusion to be established has been assumed. Thus the defender of the natural law argument is faced with a dilemma. If the law of self-preservation is said to be a law in the descriptive sense, it is surely false; and if it is said to be a law in the prescriptive sense, then the argument begs the question. Either way, the argument fails.

Let us consider another argument that might be given to show that suicide is wrong (and hence voluntary euthanasia is wrong). Often arguments against suicide try to show that there is a duty to oneself not to take one's own life. However, the notion of a duty to the self is very controversial; some philosophers argue that there can be no such thing as a duty to oneself. The argument to be considered here, though, tries to show that an individual has a duty to *others* not to commit suicide. Put simply, the argument appeals to the harm principle. It says that a person who commits suicide is harming others and so the action is wrong. How is the person who commits suicide harming others? If there are dependents, their well-being will be jeopardized. The self-inflicted death may cause family members to be unhappy and, perhaps, to feel shame. The person's suicide might also deprive others of services that he or she might have rendered or owed them. Certainly it seems plausible to restrict a person's action if it threatens to do harm to others. So if committing suicide will harm others, then there are grounds for saying that the action is wrong and may be prohibited.

But is this a good argument? There are two significant criticisms of it. First, it surely does not show that suicide is always wrong. There will be some cases where a person's committing suicide will not harm others. The self-inflicted death of the proverbial hermit will deprive no other person of services and will cause no one else to be unhappy. And there undoubtedly will be others cases too. But the second criticism is more telling. The concept of harm must be examined. If a person commits suicide, does he or she really *harm* those family members who feel hurt, ashamed, or abandoned? It is not obvious that the person does harm them. Suppose that my neighbor is a member of a conservative religious cult. Members of this cult believe that drinking alcoholic beverages is a sin. My neighbor becomes extremely upset whenever he or she sees a person consuming alcohol. If I sit on my porch and drink beer, am I harming my neighbor simply because he or she becomes upset? Surely I am not harming him. Similarly I am not harming my parents if they become extremely upset because I am living with a person of the opposite sex out of wedlock or because I refuse to have my newborn child baptized. Thus, the mere fact that an action adversely affects others does not mean that those others have been harmed. And the shame or unhappiness that friends and family members experience because of a suicide appear similar to the feelings of my neighbor or my parents. To be sure, in *some* cases a suicide will harm others. If a person jumps from the top floor of a building and lands on another person, if a person uses explosives to commit suicide and in so doing injures another, those actions would be wrong according to the harm principle. And perhaps a parent who commits suicide and leaves children as survivors who will not be cared for adequately has also harmed others. But the point is that once we reflect on the concept of harm we can see that far fewer suicides will be wrong than the proponent of the second argument against suicide believes. Certainly not all suicides will be wrong.

The proponent of voluntary euthanasia, then, can claim plausibly that the arguments (considered here) to show that suicide is always wrong fail. But can any reasons to convince us that suicide is sometimes permissible be provided? The usual strategy here is to appeal to examples. Cases are presented in which most will agree that suicide is acceptable. Consider the familiar story of Captain Oates. Oates was a member of Robert Scott's expedition to the South Pole. As he and several of his companions were returning from a mission of exploration, Oates had a serious accident and was disabled. The group was far from the depot, which was their only source of food and shelter. It appeared to each of them that if the others continued to help Oates, none would make it back alive. However, if Oates were to detach himself from the group (an act that would insure a quick death for him), the others would have a good chance to return safely. Is Captain Oates permitted to commit suicide? Surely he is. Oates has good reason to believe that no matter what he does he will die sooon. If he detaches himself from the group, that, in effect, is suicide. But if he remains with the group he will hinder their progress and all will die. Since Oates will die soon no matter what he does and since he can save several lives if he commits suicide, surely he is at least permitted to end his own life. It might even be argued that he is morally required to commit suicide. This stronger claim is controversial, however, because some say that his ending his life in order to save the others is a supererogatory act, an act above and beyond the call of duty. But whether the act is obligatory or supererogatory, it is surely at least permissible.

Consider a second case designed to show that suicide is sometimes permissible. The plane of an Army pilot goes out of control over a heavily populated area. The pilot can either bail out and let the plane fall, thereby possibly killing many civilians, or can crash-land in an area where no one else will be hurt, but by doing so will insure the pilot's own death. If the latter course of action is taken, the pilot will be bringing about his or her own death. Yet surely such an act is permissible; some would even consider it supererogatory. It is less plausible to say that the pilot is required to make this sacrifice than it is to say that Oates is so required—the reason being that Oates is going to die soon no matter what he does, but if the Army pilot bails out, he or she will presumably live for a long time.

These two cases show that sacrificing one's own life for the good of others is sometimes justified. But some have wondered whether these are really cases of committing suicide. Perhaps it is simple-minded to equate sacrificing one's own life with committing suicide. Certainly it has been said that the act of Captain Oates was not one of suicide; rather the blizzard killed him.[20] Surely, though, there are paradigmatic cases of suicide that are justified. Consider the classic case of a spy or a war criminal who has been captured by the enemy. This person knows many important secrets about our military operations and if the enemy obtains this information thousands of innocent lives will be endangered. Our spy also knows that he will be tortured and forced to reveal the information. So in order to protect the lives of those innocent persons, he or she takes a cyanide tablet and dies instantly. This is uncontroversially a case of suicide, and most will agree that the spy is justified in committing the act.

What has been shown, then, is that the objection that voluntary euthanasia is always wrong because suicide is always wrong is not convincing. Not only are the arguments to show that suicide is always wrong inadequate, but there are positive reasons to believe that suicide is at least sometimes permissible. But this, of course, does not show that voluntary euthanasia is permissible. It only shows that a standard objection to voluntary euthanasia is inadequate. And since voluntary euthanasia involves a second party bringing about a person's death while suicide only involves the victim, there may well be additional objections to the practice of euthanasia. It is worth noting that this consideration suggests that if possible it is morally preferable to allow a patient to commit suicide rather than to engage in mercy killing. The reason for this is that all but the extremists will grant that suicide is less problematic than mercy killing. That is, even those who oppose suicide will surely concede that suicide is less problematic, from the moral point of view, than a person being killed by someone else. Thus a society considering legalizing voluntary euthanasia is well-advised to opt for a program of supervised suicide, as it were, whenever possible.

But in some cases where a person wishes to be mercy killed the person is not able to perform the act alone. What sort of objections might be raised against permitting such a person to be mercy killed? Some opponents might invoke the wedge argument against the practice. Yet, such an argument is plausible only if its proponent produces evidence to show that initiating the practice will actually cause other morally undesirable practices to occur. Until such evidence is forthcoming, the wedge argument will be set aside. It must be kept in mind, however, that this argument should be examined more thoroughly. There is another objection, though, that must be considered. As previously stated, in some cases where euthanasia is requested, a second party must be the instrument of the death. For example, the person who wishes to be mercy killed may be paralyzed or may lapse into a coma after making the request. This would require someone else to be the agent of death. And typically this second party will be a medical worker. It is precisely because of the role that the nurse or physician must play that some have objected to voluntary euthanasia. Critics argue that physicians and nurses are required to preserve the lives of their patients at all costs. In particular, they claim that the codes of ethics to which these medical professionals are committed forbid at least active euthanasia. For example, the Hippocratic Oath says, "I will neither give a deadly drug to anybody if asked for it, nor will I make a suggestion to this effect." And the International Code of Nursing Ethics states that a nurse's fundamental responsibility is to conserve life. So, the critic concludes, medical professionals are forbidden to assist the patient in an act of mercy killing. There is a response to this objection, however. Professional codes of ethics are notoriously oversimplified. It is true that the Hippocratic Oath directs physicians not to participate in euthanasia. But doctors are also required by the Hippocratic Oath to benefit the sick to the best of their ability. What is a physician supposed to do if he or she judges that the best way to benefit a patient with throat cancer is to end the patient's life upon request? It is also true that the first clause of the International Code of Nursing Ethics states that the nurse is to conserve life. But there is more to the clause than that. What it actually states is this: "The fundamental responsibility of the nurse is threefold: to conserve life, to alleviate suffering, and to promote health." Now obviously the obligation to conserve life can conflict with the obligation to alleviate suffering in certain situations. In some cases the only way to ease a patient's suffering is to administer a drug so powerful that it is known it will be lethal. What is a nurse required to do when such a conflict arises? Professional codes of ethics are important and sometimes can be useful. But their value is limited. They must be oversimplified; authors of such codes cannot anticipate every kind of moral situation that might arise for the professional in question. And almost invariably there are possible circumstances in which parts of the code will conflict. It is not very convincing, then, if a critic of voluntary euthanasia rests his entire case on the fact that such an activity is proscribed by certain codes of ethics. If the code of ethics requires the medical worker to relieve suffering, as most do, there will be a conflict the resolution of which is not obvious.

Some who are not necessarily opposed to euthanasia have argued that there is no need to legalize such a practice. They support this claim by pointing out that doctors and nurses already perform acts of mercy killing. Why not leave well enough alone, they ask? It is no doubt true that medical workers often hasten the death of a terminally ill patient upon his or her request. But that is surely not an adequate reason to refrain from making such a practice legal. In particular, two points must be noted. First, there are still many doctors and nurses who will not engage in any form of euthanasia, for religious, moral, or perhaps legal reasons. If euthanasia is desirable or if the patient has a right to euthanasia upon request, then society should legalize the practice. As things stand now euthanasia occurs "underground," as it were, and only if the physician or nurse is willing to go along. Second, it is unfair to expect members of the medical profession to jeopardize their careers and risk being imprisoned simply because society in general does not want to bother legalizing euthanasia. Again, if the practice is desirable, it should be legalized.

When people are discussing the issue of euthanasia, it is often asserted that there is no moral difference between active euthanasia and passive euthanasia. It is worth exploring this claim briefly. To say that there is never a morally relevant difference between active and passive euthanasia is as misguided as the claim that active euthanasia is always worse than passive euthanasia. In particular, one factor will be cited to show that there is sometimes a morally relevant difference between the two. Medical judgments, it is clear, are not infallible. On some occasions patients live much longer than members of the medical team had predicted. Recall the recent case of Karen Quinlan. It was believed that she would die immediately after she was removed from the respirator. Yet four years later she still lives. The importance of this fallibility is this: to engage in active euthanasia removes all possibility of life for the patient; it allows no way of checking the accuracy of the judgment that the patient would have died soon anyway. But to engage in passive euthanasia—to cease extraordinary treatment—need not remove the possibility of life; if the judgment that the patient is terminally ill is wrong, passive euthanasia provides a check of sorts. This does not mean, however, that passive euthanasia is always preferable to active euthanasia. At most it suggests that passive euthanasia is preferable in those cases where the purpose of euthanasia is to end a meaningless existence, such as that of a person in an irreversible coma. But in some cases the purpose of euthanasia is to prevent needless suffering, such as the case of the person with throat cancer. Here passive euthanasia will not achieve that purpose. Thus if euthanasia is desirable in this latter sort of case, active euthanasia will be preferable to passive euthanasia. In any case, though, it seems clear that there is at least sometimes a morally relevant difference between active euthanasia and passive euthanasia.

Finally, consider an argument which purports to show that voluntary euthanasia is not wrong in certain circumstances. The argument is predicated on the assumption that each person has the right to life. Here this right is negatively construed; that is, the right to life is the right not to be killed unjustly. This argument also assumes a corollary to the right to life: each person has the right to choose whether to live or die. This is an antipaternalistic assumption, an assumption that each person has a right to autonomy. Now consider the following argument:

1. To possess a right is to possess something that constitutes a legitimate restraint on the freedom of actions of others.
2. Each person has the right to choose whether to live or to die provided that that choice does not interfere with the rights of other persons.
3. Therefore others may not interfere when a person chooses to die, provided that that choice does not interfere with anyone's rights.

Premise (1) of this argument is simply a partial analysis of what it means for a person to have a right. Premise (2) states the assumption concerning the right to life and the right to self-determination. And line (3), which follows from (1) and (2), says that it is wrong not to let a person die if he or she has freely chosen to do so. Thus *voluntary passive euthanasia* is *morally required*. That is, if a person has asked that his or her life not be saved, it would be wrong to interfere. This conclusion, though, should not be particularly surprising. Notice that this is nothing more than a case of a competent adult refusing lifesaving therapy, and there are good reasons for saying that persons do have this right. The argument can be extended in a more controversial direction, however, if the following premise is accepted.

4. Others may aid a person in exercising his or her rights if they are asked to do so and choose to comply.

With this premise added, one can derive

5. Therefore others may aid a person in exercising his or her right to carry out the choice to die if asked to do so.

Premise (4) seems simple enough. It says that a person who has a right is permitted to enlist the aid of others in exercising that right. Line (5), which follows from premises (2) and (4), says, in effect, that *voluntary active euthanasia* is morally *permissible*. If a person asks you to help him or her carry out the right to die by providing a lethal drug, you are permitted to do so. It would not be plausible to say that a person is morally required to help another exercise this right (unless, perhaps, extreme circumstances apply), but a person is allowed to do so.

Several points concerning this argument should be clarified. First, if the argument is correct, it shows that in the same situation active euthanasia and passive euthanasia can have different moral statuses. If a person asks you to help carry out the right to die, you are required not to save that person against his or her will, but assisting the person to carry out the act is merely permissible. A second point worth noting is a possibly objectionable implication of this argument. The assumptions about the right to life and the right to self-determination imply that suicide is wrong only if it interferes with the rights of others. Some will find this consequence unacceptable. Note, however, that even if suicide is permissible, it may not be rational. Even if committing suicide would not violate the rights of others, it still might be an irrational act. Some, of course, hold that both euthanasia and suicide are wrong because matters of life and death are "God's work." This assumption will not be discussed here except to point out that it also seems to imply that all forms of medical practice are wrong. If matters of life and death are "God's work," then saving lives will also constitute an interference, and few are willing to say that saving human lives is wrong.

Finally, some may hold that the right to life is construed too weakly here. The right to life, it may be argued, is a positive right. If it is construed positively, the right to life will give a person a right against others that they *save* him or her whenever possible. But even if the right to life is taken to be a positive right and if the corollary, the right to self-determination, is also accepted, voluntary euthanasia will not be wrong. In fact, taking these rights to be positive rights produces some unexpected results. If a person wants to exercise the right to die, then not only is another permitted to help, that person is actually required to help. That is, if these rights are positive rights and a person asks you to help him or her carry out the right to die, you will be required to do so. Thus voluntary active euthanasia will be morally required. This seems much too strong and suggests that the critic will not want to object to the above argument because the right to life is construed too weakly.

Another move the critic might make, of course, is to claim that there is no right to self-determination. But what reasons are there to deny that there is such a right? Certainly a plausible explanation of why slavery, coercion, kidnapping, and rape are wrong is that such actions deny a person his or her right to self-determination. If the right to autonomy or self-determination is taken seriously, it seems to follow that, minimally, voluntary passive euthanasia is required. Whether voluntary active euthanasia is permissible, however, is another matter. To reach that conclusion, at least in the argument sketched above, premise (4) must be accepted. This premise says that a person may always enlist the help of others in exercising a right. This, however, is debatable. Not all rights are like this. In virtue of being married a wife or husband may have certain rights. It surely does not follow, though, that a spouse may always ask others to help him or her exercise such rights. Whether the right to end one's life is a right that a person may enlist the help of others in exercising, then, is arguable.

## SUMMARY

To summarize this chapter completely is not possible. However, some of the highlights will be noted. It is important, for moral purposes, to distinguish between infant euthanasia and adult euthanasia. This is so because in the former case, but not the latter, the direct consent of the person whose death is induced cannot be obtained. The question of infant euthanasia arises most naturally when the child is severely deformed and has no chance of living a normal, pleasant life. There are three responses that can be made to such children: they might be killed; medical workers might do all they can to save them; or these children might be left to die. Infant euthanasia unveils a difficult moral problem because there seems to be something wrong with each of these policies.

Adult euthanasia is sometimes entertained as an option in the following situations: when a person is terminally ill and in great pain; when a person is in an irreversible coma; or when a person is suffering from severe senility or is severely retarded. Two distinctions are thought by many to carry a great deal of moral weight: the distinction between active euthanasia and passive euthanasia, and the distinction between voluntary euthanasia and involuntary euthanasia. Voluntary passive euthanasia is said to be the practice easiest to justify, while involuntary active euthanasia is the most difficult. It does not seem promising, however, to try to formulate any general rules in light of these distinctions. If only passive euthanasia is permitted, then those suffering from a terminal, painful illness may not be mercy killed. And if only voluntary euthanasia is permitted, those in an irreversible coma may not be mercy killed (unless they have explicitly expressed their wishes in advance).

At the end of the chapter an argument was sketched, an argument predicated on the assumption that each person has a strong right to self-determination. First, it was shown that voluntary passive euthanasia is morally required; that is, if a person asks that lifesaving therapy not be initiated, those wishes must be honored. Second, it was shown that voluntary active euthanasia is permissible; that is, if a person asks another for assistance in hastening his or her own death, the other person may provide this help. There are some possibly objectionable consequences of this argument, and they were noted at the end.

## CASE STUDY—1

Kenneth Wright, a former high school football star, was 24 years old. He had broken his neck in June, 1979, and had been confined to a wheelchair ever since. Before this confinement he was very active, enjoying such activities as football, hunting, skin diving, and wrestling. It seemed that he could not cope with his paralysis. On September 27, 1980, Wright was allegedly carried by two of his friends, William King and Brian Taylor, into the woods. After the friends had left, Wright killed himself with a shotgun. The laws of Connecticut (the state in which this occurred) forbid one to aid another person to commit suicide. Thus Harold Dean, the Assistant State's Attorney, charged King and Taylor with second-degree manslaughter.

### Discussion Questions

1. From the facts presented, does it seem to you that Kenneth Wright had good reasons for ending his own life? Explain why or why not.
2. Assume for the moment that Kenneth Wright had the right to commit suicide. Is this a case where it is appropriate for others to help him carry out this right? Were the actions of William King and Brian Taylor justifiable?
3. Is Connecticut's law making it illegal to help another to commit suicide justifiable? If so, how would you justify it? If not, what is wrong with it?
4. Harold Dean, the Assistant State's Attorney, stated that King and Taylor were not criminals. He said he believed that they were moved by compassion. Nevertheless he brought charges against them. Given his belief, should he have done this?

## CASE STUDY—2

In April, 1975, Karen Quinlan attended a party. After a few drinks, she passed out. Her friends put her to bed. When they checked on her, she was not breathing. They gave her mouth-to-mouth resuscitation and rushed her to the nearest hospital. Karen had not consumed a dangerous amount of alcohol and although she had taken aspirin and Valium, what caused her to stop breathing is unknown. During that time, however, part of her brain died from a lack of oxygen.

For the first three months after this incident, Karen was breathing by means of a respirator; and she was comatose. At first her parents, Joseph and Julie Quinlan, held out hope that she might recover. Doctors convinced them, however, that because of the extensive brain damage, Karen could never return to normalcy. So after Karen had been unconscious for over three months, the Quinlans gave the doctors permission to take Karen off the respirator. Surprisingly, however, the doctors refused to disconnect Karen. The Quinlans then took legal action. Since Karen was twenty-one, they had to request that the court appoint them as her legal guardians. Before the New Jersey Superior Court, they argued that the right to privacy and the right to religious freedom were at stake. Her parents also presented evidence to show that Karen would not have wanted to be kept alive artificially. In addition, they pointed out that they had no financial motive for having the respirator removed; Medicare was paying a substantial amount of the bill. Nonetheless, Judge Robert Muir ruled against them (November, 1975). They appealed the decision to the New Jersey Supreme Court, and in March, 1976, the decision was reversed and the Quinlans were permitted to have the respirator disconnected.

Karen was moved to a nursing home, where she still resides. She remains in a coma. She receives intravenous feedings and periodic doses of antibiotics to protect her against infections.

## Discussion Questions

1. Do you agree with the decision of Joseph and Julie Quinlan to have Karen's respirator removed? Explain why or why not.
2. The New Jersey Superior Court denied the Quinlans' request to be appointed the legal guardians of their 21-year-old daughter. The New Jersey Supreme Court reversed this decision. With which of these courts do you agree?
3. Karen Quinlan's respirator was removed but she continues to be fed intravenously and to be given antibiotics. Is this a reasonable policy? Is there a relevant difference between these forms of treatment?

4. Would you favor active euthanasia for Karen Quinlan? Explain why or why not.

## SUGGESTIONS FOR FUTHER READING

Mary Rose Barrington, "Apologia for Suicide," in Samuel Gorovitz *et al.* (eds.), *Moral Problems in Medicine* (Englewood Cliffs, New Jersey: Prentice-Hall, 1976), pp. 396-401.
Tom L. Beauchamp, "Suicide," in Tom Reagan (ed.), *Matters of Life and Death* (New York: Random House, 1980), pp. 67-108.
John A. Behnke and Sissela Bok (eds.), *The Dilemmas of Euthanasia* (Garden City, New York: Anchor Press, 1975).
Joel Feinberg, "Voluntary Euthanasia and the Inalienable Right to Life," *Philosophy & Public Affairs*, Vol. 7 (1978), pp. 93-123.
Philippa Foot, "Euthansia," *Philosophy & Public Affairs*, Vol. 6 (1977), pp. 85-112.
Jonathan Glover, *Causing Death and Saving Lives* (New York: Penguin Books, 1977), pp. 170-202.
Germain Grisez and Joseph M. Boyle, Jr., *Life and Death with Liberty and Justice* (Notre Dame, Indiana: University of Notre Dame Press, 1979).
Marvin Kohl (ed.), *Beneficient Euthanasia* (Buffalo, New York: Prometheus Books, 1975).
James Rachels, "Euthansia," in Tom Reagan (ed.), *Matters of Life and Death* (New York: Random House, 1980), pp. 28-66.
Bonnie Steinbock (ed.), *Killing and Letting Die* (Englewood Cliffs, New Jersey: Prentice-Hall, 1980).

## NOTES

1. I ignore here two other moral categories of actions, namely, the supererogatory and the offensive. A supererogatory action is one that is above and beyond the call of duty; it is morally desirable but not required. An offensive act is one that is undesirable but not forbidden.
2. I say *merely* permissible to distinguish this class of actions from those that are morally required. Clearly actions that are morally required are also permissible, though we would not say that they are merely permissible.
3. These examples are borrowed, with slight modifications, from James Rachels, "Active and Passive Euthanasia," *The New England Journal of Medicine*, Vol. 292 (1975), pp. 78-80.
4. These examples are presented by Gilbert Harman, *The Nature of Morality* (New York: Oxford University Press, 1977), pp. 3-4.
5. It might be suggested that there is another important difference between these two cases. A person might be said to own his or her body and the organs therein. Taking the organs without permission, therefore, would be wrong—a violation of a person's property rights. But a patient coming to the emergency room cannot be said to own the physician nor the resources to be used by the

physician. This, then, accounts for our different judgments in the two cases. Even if this is correct, the other examples show that thesis (II) is doubtful. I leave it to the reader to decide about this additional matter, however.

6. For a discussion of this point, see Philippa Foot, "The Problem of Abortion and the Doctrine of Double Effect," in Samuel Gorovitz *et al.* (eds.), *Moral Problems in Medicine* (Englewood Cliffs, New Jersey: Prentice-Hall, 1976), pp. 268-269.

7. See Foot, "The Problem of Abortion and the Doctrine of Double Effect," pp. 267-276.

8. See, for example, Bruce Russell, "On the Relative Strictness of Positive and Negative Duties," *American Philosophical Quarterly*, Vol. 14 (1977), pp. 87-97.

9. Quoted in James Rachels, "Active and Passive Euthanasia," pp. 78-80.

10. See "New Jersey Supreme Court: In the Matter of Karen Quinlan," in Tom L. Beauchamp and LeRoy Walters (eds.), *Contemporary Issues in Bioethics* (Encino, Calif.: Dickenson Publishing Company, 1978), pp. 336-346.

11. A proposal submitted by Walter Sackett to the Florida House of Representatives, however, appears to be an exception to this. Section 3 of this proposal seems to allow for involuntary euthanasia. See Walter Sackett, "An Act Relating to the Right to Die With Dignity," in Thomas A. Mappes and Jane S. Zembaty (ed.), *Social Ethics* (New York: McGraw-Hill Book Company, 1977), pp. 43-44.

12. Recently, however, a different strategy has been adopted. It has been argued that voluntary euthanasia may be permissible even if the right to life is inalienable. See Joel Feinberg, "Voluntary Euthanasia and the Inalienable Right to Life," *Philosophy & Public Affairs*, Vol. 7 (1978), pp. 93-123.

13. My discussion of the wedge argument is very superficial. For a more detailed discussion and defense of this argument, see Germain Grisez and Josephy M. M. Boyle, Jr., *Life and Death with Liberty and Justice* (Notre Dame, Indiana: University of Notre Dame Press, 1979), pp. 173-176.

14. See Robert M. Veatch, *Case Studies in Medical Ethics*, pp. 85-86.

15. Ian G. Wickes, "Ethical and Social Aspects of Treatment of Spina Bifida," in *Moral Problems in Medicine*, p. 349.

16. L. Haas, "Ethical and Social Aspects of Treatment of Spina Bifida," in *Moral Problems in Medicine*, p. 351.

17. Eliot Slater, "Health Service or Sickness Service?" in *Moral Problems in Medicine*, p. 353.

18. Those who are interested in pursuing the issue of infant euthanasia in more detail are advised to read Richard M. Hare's "Survival of the Weakest" and Derek Parfit's "Rights, Interests, and Possible People," in *Moral Problems in Medicine*, pp. 364-369 and pp. 369-375.

19. For an explanation of the naturalistic fallacy, see William K. Frankena, *Ethics* (Englewood Cliffs, New Jersey: Prentice-Hall, second edition, 1973), pp. 99-100.

20. For an excellent discussion of this issue, see Tom L. Beauchamp, "Suicide," in Tom Reagan (editor), *Matters of Life and Death* (New York: Random House, 1980), pp. 76-77.

# 6

# Abortion

When the female reproductive cell, the ovum, is fertilized by the male sex cell, the spermatozoon, the product is called the single-cell zygote. Within the first day of conception the zygote begins to divide. By the third day it consists of sixteen cells. As the zygote continues to grow during the first week, it moves through the fallopian tube into the uterus. At this point, as the zygote is gradually implanted in the uterine wall, the product of conception is called the conceptus. From the second through the eighth week of growth, it is called the embryo. From the third month until birth, it is called the fetus. In ordinary discourse, the term "fetus" is often used to refer to the product of conception at any stage of development. When the fetus is capable of living independently of the womb, it is said to be viable.

When the product of conception is expelled from the uterus prematurely, this is called abortion. When this expulsion is natural rather than intentional, it is called spontaneous abortion (or more commonly, a miscarriage). There are several different methods of performing nonspontaneous (intentional) abortions. One method, called dilation and curettage (D. and C.), involves the following: the womb is dilated and a curette is used to remove the contents of the uterus, either wholly or in pieces. A second method, suction abortion, is when the products of conception are removed from the uterus by a device that sucks the conceptus from the womb. A third method of abortion involves the injection of a saline solution into the sac containing the amniotic fluid that surrounds the conceptus; such an act induces labor. Since nonspontaneous abortion normally ends the life of a creature that is biologically human (that is, it has the same genetic code as any member of the species *Homo sapiens*), many questions have been raised about the permissibility of such a procedure.

## THE MORAL ISSUE

At what point of fetal development (if any) and for what reasons (if any) is abortion morally permissible?[1] Putting the question in this way is quite useful because it accurately suggests that there are two basic issues at the heart of the debate about abortion. The first of these two basic issues concerns the stage of fetal development. Many hold that the stage of fetal development is a morally relevant factor in determining the permissibility of abortion. The standard view, of course, is that later abortions are more morally problematic than early abortions. The second basic issue in the debate about abortion concerns the reason the woman expresses for wanting the abortion. Some reasons seem to be more acceptable than others.

Why do people disagree so radically concerning the question of abortion? Opponents in the abortion debate usually disagree about the moral status of the fetus. They disagree about whether the fetus has any rights, and if so, at what stage it has those rights. Conservatives hold that the fetus has full moral rights from the moment of conception. According to the conservative, then, the fetus has the right to life. There is, therefore, a presumption that killing the fetus is wrong. By contrast, liberals contend that the fetus has no moral status. According to this position the fetus has none of the rights that adult human beings possess. The fetus is just another piece of tissue in the woman's body. Thus a person who assents to the liberal position holds that removing the fetus is no more morally objectionable than removing the appendix. Moderates hold a position between these two extremes. They often claim that in the early stages of pregnancy the fetus does not possess full moral rights, but in the later stages it does. Thus at some point in its continuous development the fetus becomes a being with full moral rights. The moral status of the fetus, then, is one of the major sources of controversy in the debate about abortion.

Even among those who agree that abortion is at least sometimes permissible, there is considerable disagreement about what reasons justify an abortion. Let us note the reasons that have been advanced to justify abortion. It will be obvious that some of these reasons are accepted by most, while others have been advanced by only a few. The most common justification for abortion is purely medical: if the fetus is allowed to develop normally and come to term, the woman will die. Only a few would dispute that this is an acceptable reason for a woman to have an abortion. A second and related reason to justify abortion is to protect the woman's physical or mental health. Here, it is not expected that the woman will die, but carrying the fetus to full term will entail a great physical and/or mental sacrifice. That the pregnancy will produce a severely deformed child is a third reason sometimes given to justify abortion. Advocates of this reason appeal to the interests of both the parents and the fetus itself to justify abortion. Abortions performed for any of these first three reasons are often referred to as *therapeutic* abortions. This indicates, of course, that the abortion is done strictly for medical reasons.

Occasionally pregnancy is the result of rape. To force the woman to carry the fetus to full term in this case strikes many as unfair, and this is a fourth reason given to justify abortion. Some regard this as a therapeutic abortion, but since it need not be done for a purely medical reason that term will be reserved to cover only abortions performed for the first three reasons. Of course, in some cases a woman may have a medical reason for seeking an abortion after she has been raped; but many will say that she is justified in having an abortion in such cases even if it is not medically necessary. A fifth reason given to justify abortion is that the pregnancy is unwanted and therefore it saves the would-be child from an unhappy life. This reason is utilitarian in nature, purporting that abortion in certain circumstances will reduce unhappiness in the world. A sixth reason sometimes cited to justify abortion is that another child will place an unbearable financial burden on the woman or her family. This reason appeals to the consequences but is not necessarily utilitarian. It is not claimed that the *overall* unhappiness in the world will be reduced; rather it is asserted that the members of the family will be better off if abortion is performed. A seventh reason cited to justify abortion is a utilitarian one: abortion promotes a goal that is desirable in most societies, birth, or population, control. Population control, it is thought, will reduce significantly the overall suffering and unhappiness in the world. An eighth reason cited to justify abortion is relatively new.[2] Amniocentesis is the process of removing and analyzing the amniotic fluid surrounding the fetus. This process is normally used to test for potential birth defects; however, it will also reveal the sex of the fetus. Some couples want very much to have a child of a particular sex. Thus some have sought abortions because the fetus is not the preferred sex. This is a consequentialist but not a utilitarian reason; it appeals to the happiness of the couple, not to the overall happiness.

Each of the eight reasons just discussed will justify abortion only in certain situations; that is, even if these reasons are accepted, abortion will be justified only if certain conditions obtain. Some people, however, wish to opt for a much more liberal policy. They cite as a justification for abortion a ninth reason: since people have the right to do with their bodies whatever they wish, a woman may have an abortion for any reason. This justification, of course, is acceptable only to a few. It gives a woman a blank check on the question of abortion; she may obtain an abortion any time she wishes. If this justification for abortion is accepted, the other reasons become superfluous.

## ABORTION AND THE LAW

In January, 1973, the United States Supreme Court ruled on the question of abortion. Their ruling declared the restrictive abortion laws of Texas and Georgia unconstitutional. The Texas case, *Roe v. Wade*, dealt with a law that permitted abortion only when it was necessary to save the woman's life. The Georgia case, *Doe v. Bolton*, concerned a statute that allowed abortions only when it was necessary to protect the woman's health, to prevent the birth of a deformed child, or when the pregnancy resulted from rape. Each of these state laws limited a woman's right to have an abortion, though the Texas law was clearly the more restrictive of the two. Using the fictitious name of Jane Roe, a pregnant single woman challenged the constitutionality of the Texas statute. The pseudonym Jane Doe was used by the woman challenging the Georgia law. In declaring these laws unconstitutional and in stating its position on the issue of abortion, the Court appealed to three notions: the woman's right to privacy, the health of the woman, and the potential life of the fetus. Let us examine the role played by each of the concepts in the 1973 decisions.

The Court ruled that the Texas and Georgia statutes violated a woman's right to privacy, a right guaranteed by the Fourteenth Amendment. The right to privacy, the Court argued, is broad enough to encompass a woman's decision whether or not to terminate her pregnancy. Why did the Court appeal to the right of privacy in rendering its decision on abortion? Presumably they reasoned that a woman has a right to do what she wishes as long as other persons are not involved. Thus because of her right to privacy, it is the woman's choice to decide whether or not to terminate pregnancy. Such reasoning, of course, is predicated on the assumption that the fetus is not a person; apparently the fetus is regarded as just another part of the woman's body. In fact, Justice Blackmun (author of the majority opinion in *Roe v. Wade*) suggests that if the fetus were a person, then its right to life would be guaranteed by the Fourteenth Amendment and abortion would be illegal.

Why does the Court assume that the fetus is not a person? Blackmun's opinion contains two comments about the personhood of the fetus. First, Blackmun suggests that since the experts in the fields of medicine, philosophy, and theology do not agree on the question of when a being becomes a person (or, as Blackmun puts it, of when *life* begins), the judiciary cannot be expected to settle the matter. This comment reveals a skeptical attitude about the prospects of determining when personhood begins. The second comment concerns how the fetus has been regarded by the law in the past. It is claimed that no cases can be cited in which the fetus has been regarded as a person within the meaning of the Fourteenth Amendment. For example, a fetus has no property rights and must be born alive to be considered an heir. Put another way, "the unborn have never been recognized in the law as persons in the whole sense."

These two comments about the personhood of the fetus are designed to forestall the objection that all cases of abortion are wrong because it involves killing a person. It is not clear, however, that these comments succeed in accomplishing this goal. Considering the first comment, suppose that it cannot be determined whether the fetus is a person. It does not follow from this that legislation that assumes that the fetus is not a person is justified. Skepticism about the personhood of the fetus is one thing; assuming that the fetus is not a person is quite another. In short, there is a significant difference between the following two propositions: (a) there is no evidence that the fetus is a person; and (b) there is evidence that the fetus is not a person. Claim (b) is much stronger than claim (a). Lack of agreement among the experts in certain disciplines may lend credence to claim (a), but it certainly does not support claim (b). In some places, however, Blackmun seems to write as if he is entitled to assert claim (b). Concerning the second comment, it is no doubt true that there is no legal precedent for treating the fetus as a person. It does not follow from this, though, that a person may do anything whatsoever to a fetus. Animals are not recognized by the law as persons; yet the state may legitimately limit what its citizens may do to these creatures. There may, of course, be a plausible response to the objection that abortion is always wrong because it involves killing a person. Justice Blackmun's two comments, however, are not adequate in this regard.

Though the Court did appeal to a woman's right to privacy to strike down the restrictive abortion laws of Texas and Georgia, it did not go so far as to say that any restriction on abortion is unconstitutional; that is, the Court did not rule that abortion must be granted on demand. The woman's right to privacy, they argued, is not the only relevant consideration. The state also has a legitimate interest in protecting the health of the woman. In the first trimester of pregnancy, however, the state may not interfere at all in a woman's decision to have an abortion. A medical reason was given to support this judgment: the mortality rate for women having an abortion during the first trimester is lower than mortality in normal childbirth. However, a state may enact legislation to protect the woman's health during the second trimester of pregnancy and thereafter. As Blackmun puts it, "It follows that, from and after this point (the end of the first trimester), a State may regulate the abortion procedure to the extent that the regulation reasonably relates to the preservation and protection of maternal health." Blackmun then provides some specific examples of permissible regulation. "Examples of permissible state regulation in this area are requirements as to the qualifications of the person who is to perform the abortion; as to the licensure of that person; as to the facility in which the procedure is to be performed, that is, whether it must be a hospital or may be a clinic or some other place of less-than-hospital status; as to the licensing of the facility; and the like."[3] Put another way, since abortion is more dangerous to the woman during the later stages of pregnancy, the state may regulate and restrict abortion if the purpose is to protect her health. Such a restriction, of course, is paternalistic.

According to Blackmun, there is one other relevant factor in determining what sort of restrictive abortion laws a state may enact. The state has a legitimate interest in protecting, to use his words, "the potentiality of human life." Concerning the state's interest in potential life, it is argued that the compelling point is at viability; that is, when the fetus is able to live outside the woman's womb. Viability usually occurs at the beginning of the third trimester, or around the 28th week of pregnancy. Since, according to the Court, the state has a legitimate interest in protecting the "potentiality" of human life, it may forbid abortions during the third trimester. Blackmun puts it this way: "If the State is interested in protecting fetal life after viability, it may go so far as to proscribe abortion during that period except when it is necessary to preserve the life or health of the mother."[4] One point concerning this aspect of the Court's decision is worth noting here. Despite the Court's earlier claim to be unable to say when life or personhood begins, it appears, in effect, to have committed itself to the view that viability is just that magical point. Of course, this is not explicitly said by the Court. It talks instead about "potential" life. But this is surely a confusion. By any ordinary use of that term, the single-cell zygote is just as much a potential person as a viable fetus. It is tempting to say that for all practical purposes the Court has drawn the line for personhood at viability. Such a claim, however, is not quite accurate. If the Court had actually declared that the fetus were a person at viability, then it would be forced to say that its right to life is protected by the Fourteenth Amendment. And this would mean that all states would be required to prohibit abortion during the third trimester. What the Court actually suggests, however, is that states are permitted to proscribe abortion during the third trimester. Thus they seem to think that viability is important, but they do not actually say that it is the criterion of personhood.

Let us summarize briefly the position of the Supreme Court as indicated in its 1973 decisions. No state may enact legislation limiting a woman's right to have an abortion during the first trimester of pregnancy. During the second trimester the only restrictions that may be placed on abortion are those designed to protect the woman's health. In other words, a woman's right to privacy gives her the right to have an abortion during the second trimester of pregnancy, but the state may require that certain conditions be satisfied if those conditions are designed to protect the woman's health. Very restrictive laws are permitted during the third trimester except in those rare cases where abortion is necessary to protect the woman's life or health. Such restrictions are justified, the Court ruled, because the state has a legitimate interest in protecting "potential life."

## ABORTION: THE MORAL POSITIONS

What we shall call the conservative, radical, liberal, and moderate positions on the issue of abortion will now be explained in some detail. These are moral, not legal, positions. Using such terms may be somewhat misleading; they may have connotations not intended here. But the meaning of these terms will become clear as each position is explained. Put simply, the conservative position is that abortion is always wrong, or at least it is always wrong unless it is necessary to save the woman's life. According to the radical position, abortion is permissible at any stage of fetal development and for any reason. The radical holds that even infanticide is sometimes permissible. The moderate and liberal positions maintain places between these two extremes.

A warning is in order here. Although we shall be talking about the conservative position, the radical position, the liberal position, and the moderate position, such labels are misnomers. There is really no such thing as *the* conservative position, *the* radical position, and the like. There are many different and sometimes incompatible arguments that have been given to defend the conservative view. The same is true of the radical, liberal, and moderate positions. Representative and interesting arguments for each of these positions have been selected. It is only for stylistic simplicity that the word "the" is used to describe these positions.

In identifying the different views on the issue of abortion, a convention has been adopted that several other authors have used. The term "human being" is used to refer to any creature with a human genetic code. Thus any creature conceived by human parents is, at the moment of its conception, a human being. The term "human being," then, is a biological term. No moral conclusions follow from the fact that a being is human. By contrast, the term "person" is used in such a way that moral implications do follow. A person is a being with full moral rights; a person is a being with the same rights associated with normal adult human beings. In particular, a person is a being with the right to life. It need not follow, then, that all humans are persons. Whether fetuses are persons is an open question; whether human beings in irreversible comas are persons is also a matter for debate. And it may be the case that some persons are not human, depending on what characteristics constitute a person. Adopting this convention begs no questions on the issue of abortion. The ideal, rather, is to clarify the questions to be discussed. Much ink has been spilled in debating whether the fetus is a human being, a person, and the like. But what is crucial in all of this is what rights, if any, the fetus possesses. In terms adopted here, is the fetus a person? The positions to be discussed here have not always adopted this convention. Where necessary, the language of these positions has been altered to conform to our terminology.

## The Conservative Position[5]

The most crucial question in the abortion debate concerns how the personhood of a being is determined. The conservative deals with this question by adopting the following thesis: any being conceived by parents that are persons is itself a person. Since it is assumed that adult human beings are persons, it will follow that any being conceived by them is a person; thus the human fetus is a person. The conservative believes that if this thesis is established then abortion at any stage of fetal development is prima facie wrong. The argument to show that such a conclusion follows is a simple one.

i.    It is prima facie wrong to kill a person.
ii.   Human fetuses are persons.
iii.  Therefore it is prima facie wrong to kill human fetuses.
iv.   To abort a human fetus is (normally) to kill it.
v.    Therefore it is prima facie wrong to abort a human fetus.

This argument appears to be valid; that is, it seems that the conclusion follows from the premises. Lines (i), (ii), and (iv) are the premises of the argument. Line (iii) follows from (i) and (ii); line (v), from (iii) and (iv). If the form of this argument is correct, as it seems to be, then the critical question concerns the correctness of the three premises. Premises (i) and (iv) seem plausible. The adequacy of this argument, then, depends on the plausibility of premise (ii). The conservative's thesis—that any being conceived by persons is itself a person—will, if acceptable, establish premise (ii). Thus the conservative's task is to argue for this account of personhood. This will lend credence to premise (ii) and that, in turn, should make the conclusion acceptable.

How does the conservative try to establish this thesis? An eliminative strategy is usually adopted. That is, the conservative usually considers other criteria of personhood proposed by opponents and tries to show that these are inadequate. There is a certain danger in following this strategy. In order for it to be completely successful, all of the alternative criteria that might be proposed must be considered. It is most unlikely that this can be done. But if serious doubts are raised about the standard criteria of personhood, perhaps this will render the conservative view more plausible. Clearly, though, it will not establish the view. Even if the views of one's opponents are inadequate, it need not follow that one's own views are correct.

As will be seen, the radical holds that a human being does not obtain the characteristics that make him or her a person until sometime after birth. It might be expected that a natural place for the conservative to begin would be with the position of the radical. However, few conservatives have taken this route. Perhaps they think that the views of the radical are absurd. For whatever reason, though, it is with the criterion of birth that the conservative usually begins. Suppose that someone argues that abortion at any stage of fetal development is permissible but that infanticide is wrong. Apparently such a person takes birth to be the point at which a being gains rights, the right to life in particular. In the terms adopted earlier, birth is the point at which a human being becomes a person according to this view. The conservative attacks this criterion along the following lines. To say that a being obtains rights at birth is to draw a moral line without any basis. What is so special about birth? More to the point, there seems to be no morally relevant difference between an eight-month-old fetus and a newborn baby. To put it crudely, the only difference is one of geography and that is not morally relevant. Moreover, if birth is taken as the criterion of personhood, the following results: a prematurely born child whose biological life (that is, its life since conception) is seven months will have rights that an eight-month-old fetus does not have. This seems unacceptable. Birth does not seem to be a plausible place to mark that magical point at which a being acquires rights.

Let us turn, then, to a more moderate criterion. Viability is a popular place to draw the line for when a human fetus acquires the right to life. When the fetus is viable—when it is capable of living outside the womb—it is a person and it is wrong to kill it. As was seen earlier, the Supreme Court came close to adopting this position. Many who want to say that abortions in the later stages of pregnancy are wrong but that early abortions are permissible select viability as the criterion for personhood. What might the conservative say about this criterion? First, some conservatives have pointed out that if artificial incubation is perfected, as it probably will be, then the fetus will be viable at any time, or at least much earlier than it now is. Why is this important? It suggests that if viability is taken as the criterion of personhood, then personhood depends upon the state of technology, and nothing more. But this seems absurd. Surely when a being comes to possess full moral rights cannot depend upon the state of technology. Of course, proponents of the viability criterion may respond that they mean natural viability, not artificial incubation. But this leads to the next criticism.

Different fetuses are viable at different ages. And, it is claimed, Negroid fetuses are viable several weeks before Caucasian fetuses, on the average. Thus if viability is accepted as the criterion of personhood, different beings will acquire full moral rights at different times. Moreover, becoming a person will partly depend on race. This seems unacceptable and so further doubt is cast on viability as the criterion of personhood. There is a third and related criticism. Before the fetus is viable, it is absolutely dependent on the mother for its life. But, the conservative points out, dependence is not ended by viability. A child is dependent on others for years after its birth. It literally cannot survive if others do not tend to its needs. There is, of course, one difference: a previable fetus is dependent on one person, its mother, for survival; a postviable fetus is dependent on someone or other to nurture and care for it. But surely this difference is not great enough to justify the claim that a postviable fetus has the right to life and a previable fetus does not.

Let us consider one other criticism of viability as the criterion for personhood. There is something very strange about this criterion. The moderate who proposes it tells us that since the previable fetus is absolutely dependent on the mother for its life, it does not have full moral rights and may be aborted; since the postviable fetus is not absolutely dependent on the mother, however, it does possess the right to life and may not be aborted. But, morally speaking, this seems to reverse things. Normally dependence creates obligations. The obligations of parents toward their children are greater when the children are young and not able to fend for themselves. As the children grow older, the parents have fewer obligations. The proponent of viability as the criterion for when a being acquires the right to life, though, suggests that there are no obligations toward the fetus as long as it is absolutely dependent on its mother for life. Since this totally reverses moral considerations as we know them in other contexts, some justification might be expected. But the moderate usually offers none. For these reasons, then, the conservative rejects the criterion of viability.

Experience or simple consciousness is another criterion for when a being acquires the right to life. Some moderates on the abortion issue have proposed such a criterion. The underlying idea is that a being who is capable of having experiences, who can experience pain or pleasure, has some special claims. So, some moderates argue, simple consciousness is the point at which a human being acquires the right to life. The conservative rejects this criterion by pointing out that it may not serve the moderate in the way that is desired. Fetuses have experience as early as the eighth week, the conservative claims. The evidence cited to support this claim is that the fetus responds to touch at this stage of development. Whether this counts as having experience or being conscious is an open question. But if this is taken as evidence of consciousness, then those who adopt this criterion will have to admit that the fetus has the right to life as early as the eighth week of its development. This will make immoral many abortions that most moderates approve of.

The conservative's second point is a more direct criticism. The conservative thinks that accepting consciousness as the criterion for when a human being acquires the right to life has an implausible consequence. If this criterion is accepted, it will follow that adult human beings who are in a permanent coma will not have the right to life. Two things should be noted about this criticism. First, it is not obvious that this result does follow. The person who appeals to simple consciousness may hold the position that once a being attains consciousness, it has the right to life until it dies. Thus, even if it becomes unconscious, it still has the right to life. Second, many will not find counterintuitive the judgment that a person in a permanent coma does not have the right to life. Most conservatives on the abortion issue reject that judgment, but as was seen in the previous chapter, there are those who would advocate adult euthanasia in such cases. It seems, then, that the conservative's criticism of the criterion of simple consciousness is not very convincing.

Having supposedly eliminated the competing views, the conservative hopes that there will be a stronger inclination to accept the position that the fetus possesses the right to life from the moment of conception. However, the following objection might be raised against the conservative's view. If the single-cell zygote must be regarded as a person with the right to life, why not say that the sperm and the egg have the right to life too? In fact, does not consistency require that the conservative say this? And this is taken as a criticism because it shows that the conservative position implies an absurd result: that all forms of birth control are wrong because they deny to the sperm and the egg their right to life.[6] Some conservatives have tried to show that their position does not have this consequence.[7] They argue that drawing the line at conception is not arbitrary; that is, there is a morally relevant difference between the zygote on the one hand and the sperm and egg on the other. To convince one of this, the conservative appeals to probabilities. In a normal male ejaculation there are as many as 200 million spermatozoa, while a woman produces about 10,000 eggs in the ovaries, of which 400 are ovulated each month. The probabilities, then, that any given sperm or any given egg will grow into a reasoning, adult human being are extraordinarily low even if pregnancy occurred with each ejaculation; and happily that does not happen. So the probability that any given sperm will grow into an adult human being is considerably less than 1 in 200 million. Once a zygote is formed, though, the probability that it will grow into an adult human being is high. How high that probability is depends on the rate of spontaneous abortion. There is disagreement within the scientific community about just how high that rate is. It has been estimated as low as 15 percent and as high as 50 percent.[8] Even if the higher estimate is correct, however, the probability that any given zygote will become an adult human being is very high when compared with the probability that a sperm or an egg will become part of such a being. And, the argument goes, such a difference in probabilities makes a moral difference. If a person were to shoot into a bush and the chances were 200 million to one that in doing so another person would be killed, it is not very likely that that person would be held blameworthy. But if the chances were one in two that so shooting would kill a person, the person would be blamed for the act.

The differences in probabilities, then, make a moral difference and so the conservative need not say that either the sperm or the egg has the right to life. Moreover, the conservative points out, the zygote has a complete human genetic code while neither the sperm nor the egg does. The moral relevance of this latter consideration, however, is doubtful.

To conclude this summary of the conservative position, note what may be its more serious problems. First, as already indicated, there is a danger in employing an eliminative strategy. One never knows if all of the alternative views have been considered. And in any case, a positive argument for the thesis that the fetus is a person and so possesses moral rights from the moment of conception would be desirable. Few positive arguments have been given to support this thesis, however. Usually proponents appeal to religious considerations. God has somehow endowed these beings with the right to life. Although such religious views will not be considered here, it should be noted that it is desirable, as a matter of philosophical strategy, to build ethical positions on nonreligious grounds. The fewer assumptions that are made the better. If an appeal to religious considerations must be made in order to salvage the conservative position, this will certainly count against that position on philosophical grounds.

Second, consider the case in which a woman becomes pregnant due to rape. Most people are inclined to approve of abortion under this circumstance. Yet it seems that the conservative cannot consistently allow for this. Recall that the essence of the conservative position is that the fetus possesses the right to life, the same right to life as any other human being. Admittedly a serious wrong occurs when rape takes place. But the wrongdoing is perpetrated by the child's father, not the child. When a person does something wrong, he or she sometimes forfeits some rights. The child, however, cannot be said to have forfeited some of its rights because of the immoral actions of its father. How can the moral turpitude of the father affect the fetus's right to life? It would seem, then, that the conservative will be hard pressed to permit abortion even when the pregnancy is due to rape. The conservative must bite the bullet, it seems, and argue that the woman must make a sacrifice for the sake of the child. This is not a desirable result, but it seems to follow because the conservative stakes the whole case on the right to life of the innocent fetus.

Third, it is not entirely clear that the conservative can even allow abortion when the woman's life is at stake. To be sure, some conservatives have argued that they can consistently allow for abortion in this extreme and rare case.[9] What we have in such a situation, of course, is a conflict of rights. The right to life of the woman conflicts with the right to life of the fetus. Some conservatives have suggested that in these circumstances the woman's right to life may prevail because she has the right to defend herself. There are, however, several problems with this claim. First, even if the woman has the right to self-defense, it is not obvious that a medical practitioner may act on her behalf. Second, it is not clear that the right to self-defense is applicable here. The being that poses a threat to the woman's life is innocent and, as shall be discussed later, it is questionable whether killing an innocent threat can accurately be described as self-defense. Third, considerations of fairness may force the conservative to prefer the fetus to the woman in case of a conflict. After all, according to the conservative each is innocent and each has the right to life. Since one must be sacrificed, wouldn't a consistent conservative be required to favor the fetus since it has had no chance to experience life while the woman has lived many years? Perhaps the conservative is not committed to this judgment. But when the sole foundation of a view is based on the right to life of the fetus—a right said to be as strong as any other—the conservative at least owes us an argument on why this result can be avoided.

Finally, the conservative's argument logically requires a condemnation of at least some forms of birth control. In particular, any method of birth control that allows conception to take place and then, in effect, destroys the fertilized egg—for example, an I.U.D. (an intrauterine device)—is, according to the conservative, a form of abortion. It is destroying a being that has the right to life. Any version of the proverbial "morning after" pill should be rejected by the conservative for the same reason. Such a conclusion, though, seems quite extreme. Is using an I.U.D. really to engage in a form of impermissible killing? To say that it is stretches the moral imagination. Admittedly, many who think of themselves as conservatives are not opposed to such forms of birth control. Rather they object to most abortions that are performed in hospitals today. In these cases the fetus is usually at least six weeks old. But why do these people oppose abortions and not the use of an I.U.D.? They must hold that something of moral importance happens between conception and the sixth week of pregnancy. Perhaps they hold that implantation is morally significant. In any case, this is not the conservative position as it has been defined here; it is a version of the moderate position that will be discussed later. These four points, then, stand as difficulties that any defender of the conservative position needs to address.

## The Radical Position[10]

The radical position on the question of abortion holds that not only is abortion at any stage of fetal development and for any reason morally acceptable, but that infanticide is also permissible. The conservative holds that a human fetus and, of course, a newborn baby have the right to life. The radical disagrees with this claim. The radical agrees with the conservative that the fetus is a human being but does not agree that it is a person; that is, the radical does not agree that the fetus has a right to life. The disagreement between the conservative and the radical, then, is a moral disagreement. They disagree about what properties a thing must possess before it can be said to have a right to life.

The rights a being has depend on the properties that it possesses. If two beings possess all of the same properties, then they must possess the same rights. And even if they do not possess all of the same properties, if they possess the same *relevant* properties, they have the same rights. Consider a simple example. It is wrong to torture a human being and it is wrong to torture a kitten. Why is this wrong? If each of these creatures has the right not to be tortured, there must be some property they have in common in virtue of which they have that right. The obvious property that comes to mind here is the capacity to experience pain. It is in virtue of that property that each has the right not to be tortured.

What properties endow a being with the right to life? It is this question that the radical must answer. Rather than focusing on the areas of disagreement, perhaps we can begin with the areas of agreement between the radical and the conservative. Consider the following beings: adult human beings, infants, human fetuses, cows, pigs, and rats. All parties to the dispute agree that adult human beings possess the right to life. And, it seems, most agree that cows, pigs, and rats do not possess the right to life. At least, all of those who eat meat behave as if cows and pigs do not have the right to life. And it seems unlikely that anyone will say that rats have the right to life. This, then, will be our starting point. In determining what properties endow a being with the right to life, the question that must be asked is this: what do adult human beings possess that rats, pigs, and cows lack? Of course, not just any difference will do; there must be some reason to believe that these differentiating properties give a being, any being that has them, the right to life. The requirement of moral relevance eliminates one obvious answer that the conservative might propose: genetic code. Certainly adult human beings have a genetic code that is quite different from that of rats, pigs, and cows. But mere difference in genetic code does not constitute a moral difference. Imagine that we were to encounter a being from another planet. It is like us in that it has desires, expectations, it worries about the future, it communicates with us, and the like. It differs from us only in its genetic makeup. Surely if this is the only difference, this being has the same rights that we do.

How, then, does the radical go about answering the question of what properties are necessary to give a being the right to life? The radical will begin by stating what properties are necessary to endow a being with the right to life. In defense of this hypothesis, the radical will explain what having the right to life means, why the proposed criterion is appropriate, and why the conservative's view fails. Let us begin, then, with the hypothesis itself. The radical suggests that for a being to have a serious right to life, it must have at least the following properties: the capacity to envisage a future for itself, the capacity to have a concept of the self, and the capacity for self-consciousness.[11] A being that possesses the concept of a future for itself must now possess, or once have possessed, the capacity to understand what it would be like for it to continue to exist. It must also possess desires about its future states. A being that possesses the capacity to have a concept of the self must now possess, or once have possessed, the ability to think of itself as a continuing subject of experiences. Clearly normal adult human beings do have these three capacities. And it seems that rats, pigs, and cows lack such capacities. What about infants and human fetuses, however? Surely they do not have these capacities either. According to the radical, then, infants and human fetuses do not have a right to life. Abortion and infanticide are thus permissible.

But why should we accept the radical's claim that having the capacities for self-consciousness, to envisage a future for oneself, and to possess the concept of the self are necessary conditions for possessing the right to life? To understand why the radical thinks that this proposal is plausible, the radical's analysis of the right to life must first be understood, and before that, the radical's account of what it is for a being to possess any sort of right. If someone has a right, it puts a legitimate restriction on what others may do to him or her. More specifically, if a person has a right, then others have a prima facie obligation to act or to refrain from acting in certain ways toward that person. So far the account is the standard one. The radical, however, claims that the obligations correlative with rights are conditional. The correlative obligations are dependent on the existence of certain desires of the individual to whom the right is ascribed. If a person asks another to destroy something to which he or she would normally be said to have a (property) right, one does not violate the person's rights if one proceeds to destroy it. In effect, if a person does not desire something, that person has no right to it, or at least another who denies that person the thing in question is not violating that person's right. The radical, of course, wants to allow that a person can possess a desire for something without being constantly conscious of it. Persons who are asleep, for example, can still be said to desire that their property not be destroyed. The radical, then, suggests the following analysis of what it is for a being to possess a right: "$A$ has a right to X" means roughly "If $A$ desires X, then others under a prima facie obligation to refrain from actions that will deprive $A$ of X."[12] Such an analysis puts limits on the sort of creature that can even possess a right. To possess rights a being must not lack consciousness and must be capable of having desires. To illustrate, both human beings and kittens have a right not to be tortured, and each seems to possess the requisite desire related to this right: the desire not to experience pain.

How does the radical analyze the right to life? If a being is killed, it ceases to exist. To possess a right to life, there must at least be a desire to continue to exist. The radical then proposes the following analysis of the right to life: "Person $A$ has the right to life" means roughly "$A$ is a being that has experiences, $A$ has the capacity to desire to continue to exist as a subject of experiences, and if $A$ desires to continue to exist as a being that has experiences, others have a prima facie obligation not to prevent $A$ from so existing." A necessary condition for one's having a right to life is that one have a desire to continue to exist as a subject of experiences. The sort of creatures that can have the right to life, then, are those that must possess certain concepts. A being must be self-reflective—that is, it must possess the concept of the self and must be conscious that it does—and it must possess the concept of the future. A being must have at least this conceptual apparatus before it can desire to continue to exist as a subject of experiences. This analysis of the right to life is supposed to have independent plausibility. If to live is to continue to exist as a subject of experiences, then the analysis of the right to life should reflect this, and the radical's analysis does. The more fundamental assumption, that rights and their correlative duties are in force only when the being has the requisite desires, is an assumption that needs more defense than the radical provides.

If the radical's analysis of the right to life is correct, normal adult human beings possess that right and so it is prima facie wrong to kill them. Rats and pigs lack the appropriate properties, it seems, and so it is not prima facie wrong to kill them (or at least it is not wrong because they have the right to life). It seems clear, though, that human fetuses and newborn infants also lack these properties, and so according to the radical it is not wrong to kill them either. For this reason, of course, the conservative must reject the radical's account. The radical's account may also imply that a person in a permanent coma lacks the right to life. Such a being can no longer envisage a future for itself, no longer has the capacity to have a concept of the self, and no longer has the capacity for self-consciousness. Such a conclusion can be avoided only if the radical holds that any being that possesses or has possessed the relevant properties has the right to life thenceforth.

To complete this argument, the radical usually criticizes opponents' criteria for the point at which a being acquires the right to life. The radical does not think that the various criteria suggested by moderates are at all plausible. Criticisms of two such criteria will be considered here.[13] As was seen earlier, some take viability to be the point at which a human fetus gains the right to life. When a fetus is viable, it is able to live outside the womb; before it is viable, it is totally dependent on the woman for its survival. But why, the radical asks, should being in a state of total dependence on another deny to a creature the right to life? Consider the case of Siamese twins. If one of the twins would die were the two to be separated, then it is totally dependent on the other for its life. Yet it would be implausible to hold that this twin lacked the right to life. Viability, then, does not seem to be a defensible criterion. A second criterion suggested by some moderates is motility, the ability to move about spontaneously. Upon examination, however, motility does not seem to be an acceptable criterion for the point at which a being acquires the right to life either. It can be argued that the ability to move spontaneously is neither a necessary nor a sufficient condition for possessing the right to life. It is not a necessary condition for possessing the right to life because there are some beings who cannot move about spontaneously but who do have the right to life. A paralyzed human being satisfies this description. Motility is not a sufficient condition for a being's having the right to life because there are many beings that are capable of moving about spontaneously but which few believe have the right to life. Rats, pigs, and insects satisfy this description. Because of these considerations, then, neither viability nor motility is an appropriate property to endow a being with the right to life.

Some, of course, have suggested quickening as the point at which to draw the line. Quickening is that point at which the mother can feel the fetus moving. It is difficult to understand, though, why anyone would think that the fetus's right to life would be determined by some property of the woman. It seems more reasonable that when and whether a being possesses the right to life is determined by its own properties. Thus quickening is an even less plausible criterion than either viability or motility.

The conservative, though, proposes that human beings possess the right to life from the moment of their conception. How does the radical handle this view? The radical begins by trying to show that the conservative must accept the potentiality principle. The potentiality principle says that any organism potentially possessing a property that endows a being with the right to life has itself a serious right to life now in virtue of that potentiality. What does it mean to say that a being potentially possesses a property? An organism potentially possesses a property if it will come to have that property in the normal course of its development. That is, if no one interferes with its development, it will come to possess the property in question. The idea is this: it is known (or at least believed) that adult human beings possess the right to life. Thus there is some property or properties that adult human beings possess which gives them this right. Whatever that property is, the human fetus possesses it potentially; it will come to possess this property in the normal course of its development. If the conservative accepts the potentiality principle, it will provide grounds for saying that the human fetus, even the single-cell zygote, possesses the right to life. More importantly—and this is the first reason why the conservative should accept the potentiality principle—if the potentiality principle is accepted, the conservative can attribute to the human fetus the right to life *without specifying what properties give a being that right*. As long as others agree that adult human beings possess the right to life, then with the addition of the potentiality principle the conservative position can be established. Unlike the moderate, the liberal, or the radical, the conservative need not specify the properties that endow a being with the right to life. Philosophically, this is a great advantage.

There is a second reason why the conservative should and must accept the potentiality principle. Consider the following puzzle that opponents might present to the conservative. "You, the conservative, say that it is wrong to kill human fetuses at any point. Yet you would not say that it is wrong to kill, for example, pig fetuses, ape fetuses, or rat fetuses. Since you do not attribute the right to life to adult members of these species, you cannot plausibly say that their fetuses have this right. But what is the morally relevant difference between, say, a one-month old human fetus and a one-month old ape fetus? Regarding their mental lives, there is no difference; neither has mental states. So why is it wrong to kill one and not the other?" This presents the conservative with a challenge. The conservative must find some morally relevant difference between the human fetus and the ape fetus, and that difference cannot be found in properties they now possess. Certainly the answer suggested by common sense is that the difference is to be explained in terms of potential. There is a great difference in what these two creatures will become. In fact, that is surely the only relevant difference. Their genetic codes are different, of course, but, as was already seen, that is not a morally relevant difference. In order to provide a satisfactory solution to this puzzle, then, the conservative must accept the potentiality principle. If the potentiality principle is unacceptable, then so is the conservative position on abortion.[14]

Having shown that the conservative should and must accept the potentiality principle, the radical's strategy is to show that that principle is false. To do so, the radical must first advance the moral symmetry principle.[15] The moral symmetry principle, in effect, says that if the motivation is the same, then there is no moral difference between intentionally refraining from bringing about state of affairs $S$ and actively preventing state of affairs $S$ from occurring. Put another way, if the motivation is the same, then from the moral point of view there is no difference between the person who could have brought about $S$ but refrained from doing so and the person who actively interfered with a causal chain that would have resulted in $S$'s occurring. Similarly, the moral symmetry principle tells us that, if the motivation is the same, there is no moral difference in the action of a person who brings about state of affairs $S$ and one who refrains from preventing $S$ from occurring. Support for this principle usually comes in the form of examples. Thus one is asked to consider the following two cases. First, suppose that Jones sees that Smith will be killed by a bomb unless he warns her. But since Jones wants Smith dead, he allows her to be killed by the bomb. Second, suppose that Jones wants Smith dead and therefore shoots her. Do we think that Jones's behavior is less reprehensible in the first case than the second? We do not, the radical claims. And a plausible explanation of why we do not think there is a significant difference in the two cases is that we accept the moral symmetry principle.

Given this, the radical invites us to consider the following situation. Suppose that a special chemical with some very unusual properties were discovered. When injected into the brain of a kitten, this chemical will cause the kitten to develop into a cat which possesses the same sort of brain that human beings possess. Cats that have been injected will possess the same psychological attributes as adult human beings. These cats will be able to think, to use language, to express their desires, to indicate their worries about the future, and the like. How should such cats be treated? Concerning this hypothetical case, the radical offers the following four points.

1.  If right to life is ascribed to adult members of the species *Homo sapiens*, then consistency requires that the right to life be ascribed to cats that have undergone the process of development as a result of having been injected with the special chemical. There are no morally relevant differences between adult human beings and these special cats. There are, of course, differences in physical appearance, but such differences are not morally relevant ones.

2.  It would not be wrong to refrain from injecting a kitten with this special chemical and to kill it instead. (The idea here is that normal kittens do not have the right to life. If the reader thinks that kittens do have the right to life, let him or her select some other nonhuman animal that does not possess this right. The species used in this example is not important. What is important is that, by hypothesis, the creature can be transformed to possess the properties that endow a being with the right to life as a result of being injected with the chemical.) The mere fact that it is within our power to transform a kitten into a being that possesses the right to life does not imply that there is an obligation to do so. If a normal kitten does not possess the right to life, there is no duty to change it into a being that does have this right. If there were such an obligation, then any form of birth control would also be immoral, a view that is not very plausible.

3.  The moral symmetry principle tells us that if it is not wrong to refrain from initiating a given causal process, then it is not wrong to interfere with such a process before the end has been brought about. Thus if it is not wrong to refrain from injecting a kitten with the special chemical and to kill it instead, then it is not wrong to inject the kitten with the special chemical but kill it before it develops the properties that endow a being with the right to life. In the former case a person is refraining from initiating a certain process; in the latter case, that person is preventing the process from reaching its natural completion.

Given the moral symmetry principle and the conclusion reached in point 2, this result follows.

4. If it is not wrong to destroy an injected kitten before it develops the properties that endow a being with the right to life, then neither is it wrong to destroy a member of the species *Homo sapiens* which does not now possess those properties but which will acquire them naturally. An injected kitten and a human fetus have the same moral status: neither presently has the properties necessary to endow a being with the right to life, but each will naturally come to possess them in the process of its development. If potentiality endows a being with the right to life, both the injected kitten and the human fetus possess the right to life and it would be wrong to kill either. But, as was just seen, it is not wrong to kill an injected kitten. Therefore, it is not wrong to kill a member of the species *Homo sapiens* before it develops the properties that give a being the right to life.

The radical's argument, then, is that the conservative position is correct only if the potentiality principle is plausible. But the potentiality principle is not plausible; the hypothetical case of the special chemical that will transform a being that normally does not possess the right to life into a being that does possess this right shows this. The reader should be aware, however, that the argument of the radical presented here requires that one accept the moral symmetry principle. If the moral symmetry principle is unacceptable, this alleged refutation of the conservative position will collapse. No attempt will be made here to determine whether the moral symmetry principle is plausible. Anyone pondering this matter, though, should ask whether an agent's motivation is ever relevant to the rightness or wrongness of the ensuing actions. Defenders of the moral symmetry principle do assume that motives do affect the moral status of an action, and this is one of many assumptions that should be examined critically.

Let us review the strategy up to this point. The radical has argued that the only sort of being that possesses a right to life is one that has the capacity to envisage a future for itself, the capacity to have a concept of the self, and the capacity for self-consciousness. Adult human beings normally possess these capacities; human fetuses and newborn infants do not. The radical, then, has considered competing criteria suggested by opponents, criteria for when a being acquires a right to life. The radical has tried to show that each of these criteria is inadequate.

There is thus a positive argument and a negative argument to support the radical position.

A practical problem remains, however. At what point in time after birth does an infant acquire the capacity to envisage a future for itself, the capacity to have the concept of the self, and the capacity for self-consciousness? The answer to this question depends on work in empirical psychology. How the question is answered, however, is very important. The radical faces nothing less than the all too familiar problem of "drawing the line." If the position of the radical is correct, not only is abortion at any stage of fetal development permissible, but infanticide is also permissible. But at what point does infanticide cease to be permissible? Since there is currently no way to determine that point at which the fetus or newborn infant becomes a person, the radical offers the following suggestion. When infanticide is desirable—for example, when the infant has severe birth defects—it is usually evident in the first week after birth. Given this and our ignorance about when human beings acquire the properties that endow them with the right to life, the radical proposes a path of caution. If we err, err on the side of life. For the time being, then, the line should be drawn at the admittedly arbitrary time of one week after birth. That is, infanticide should only be permitted during the first week after birth but not thereafter. If significant advances are made in the study of infant psychology, then perhaps this line can be redrawn. But for now caution must prevail.

One other practical problem remains. It may be that adult members of other species possess the properties that endow them with the right to life. Of course, most human beings behave as if they believe that only human beings possess this right. However, this view may be mistaken. Only investigation in the area of animal psychology will provide the answer to this question. The point the radical wants to make, though, is that the rights a being possesses depends on the properties it has. Being a member of a certain species is not in itself a morally relevant characteristic. Therefore once the properties that endow a being with the right to life have been specified, the possibility that beings other than adult humans also have the right to life must be acknowledged. Which beings other than adult humans have this right is a matter to be determined by empirical investigation.

## The Liberal Position[16]

The liberal and the moderate positions differ only in degree. Each agrees that abortion is sometimes permissible and sometimes wrong.

The liberal, however, holds that abortion is permissible in certain cases and for certain reasons that the moderate will not allow. There are many different versions of the liberal position. A widely discussed version of that position will be presented here.

The conservative holds that the fetus is a person and therefore possesses a right to life from the moment of conception. The strategy of those who disagree with the conservative is usually to deny that the fetus is a person from the moment of conception. Thus, typically, the moderate, the liberal, and the radical argue that personhood is attained by human beings sometime after conception; they differ, of course, on when that point is. The liberal position to be discussed here, however, takes a different approach. It is granted to the conservative, for the sake of argument, that the fetus is a person and has the right to life from the moment of conception. Why does the conservative think that it follows from this that abortion is always wrong? Earlier a version of the conservative's argument was stated, but let us recast that argument by making the right to life a prominent part of it. This revised argument may be stated as follows: (i) Every person has the right to life. (ii) The fetus is a person (from the moment of its conception). (iii) So the fetus has the right to life. (iv) Therefore killing the fetus is wrong, and so abortion is wrong. Rather than quibble about when a being acquires the right to life, the liberal hopes to show that even if the fetus has that right, abortion is not always (or even often) wrong. If such an argument succeeds, it will be very powerful. If the most cherished premise of the conservative, that the fetus has the right to life, can be granted, and if it can still be shown that abortion is not always wrong, the conservative position will have been mortally wounded.

What the conservative supposes is that the connection between the right to life and killing is simple: if a being has the right to life, it is always wrong to kill it. It is this assumption that enables the conservative to move from (iii) to (iv) in the above argument. The liberal wants to challenge this assumption by arguing that even if a being possesses the right to life, it is not always wrong to kill it. In challenging the move from (iii) to (iv), there are at least three different approaches that the liberal might take.

The *first* approach will be called the self-defense argument. Suppose that carrying a child full term will endanger the life of the woman. The woman is a person and so she too has the right to life. And a being that has a right to life has a right to defend itself whenever its life is threatened. So, the argument goes, even if the fetus does have the right to life, the woman is permitted to abort it in order to save her own life.

This alone, of course, does not establish anything resembling a liberal position; it only shows that abortion is allowed in one sort of case. However, the self-defense argument is not designed to establish the liberal position. Its purpose is to show that the conservative's assumption that it is always wrong to kill a being which has the right to life is false.

There are some grounds for wondering, though, whether the self-defense argument achieves even its modest aim. The problem with this approach is that what constitutes self-defense is not always clear. To illustrate this point, let us consider the following three cases. (1) You kill $X$ because $X$ is trying to kill you and killing $X$ is the only way that you can prevent $X$ from killing you. (2) $X$ threatens to kill you and your two children (and $X$'s threat is credible) unless you kill $Y$, an innocent person against whom $X$ holds a grudge. (3) You just learn that someone has rigged the light switch so that when it is moved it will set off a bomb in the room you now occupy. $X$, an innocent person, is about to switch the light on and thus to detonate the bomb unwittingly. The circumstances are such that you can prevent $X$ from detonating the bomb only if you shoot $X$. If you do not shoot $X$, you will be killed.

Case (1) is a paradigmatic case of self-defense. Clearly a person is justified in killing $X$ in this case. Case (2), most agree, is not a case where a person may kill $Y$ and claim that the act was one of self-defense. It is true that $Y$'s continued existence poses a threat to the agent. But this is only because of the interference of a not-so-innocent party, $X$. What about case (3)? If the agent in this case kills $X$, is that a legitimate case of self-defense? To help us answer this question, let us ask how the unproblematic cases, cases (1) and (2), differ.

There seem to be two important differences between these two cases. First, in case (1) the person whose continued existence poses a threat to the agent's life is not an innocent party; that person is responsible for the fact that he or she is a threat to the agent. In case (2) the person whose continued existence poses a threat to the agent's life is innocent. Second, in case (1) it is the specific actions of the person whose continued existence poses a threat to the agent that will kill the agent. In case (2) though it is $Y$ whose continued existence poses a threat to the agent, it is the actions of some third party, $X$, that will kill the agent. How does case (3) fare with respect to these two characteristics? Unfortunately, in one respect it is like case (2), but in the other respect it is like case (1). Like case (2), in case (3) the party whose continued existence poses a threat to the agent is innocent. But like case (1) and unlike (2), in case (3) it is the specific actions of the person whose continued existence poses a threat to the agent that will kill the agent. Thus in one respect case (3) is like the paradigmatic case of self-defense; in another respect, it is quite unlike it.

What is the point of all of this? When a woman's reason for wanting an abortion is that the continued existence of the fetus poses a threat to her life, this is a situation that is like case (3). Clearly the fetus is an innocent party, and yet it is the action of the fetus (Is growth an action?) that will kill the woman. The point, then, is that abortion in this case, just like killing $X$ in case (3), is not an obvious case of self-defense. Whether it is a case of self-defense is problematic. This is because the concept of self-defense requires further clarification. Thus in criticizing the conservative's claim that since the fetus has the right to life it is always wrong to kill it, grounds other than self-defense should be found. For unless a person is prepared to elaborate at great lengths on the concept of self-defense, such an argument will not be totally convincing.

How else might the liberal challenge the move from (iii) to (iv) in the conservative's argument? A *second* approach appeals to the notion of a supererogatory act. A supererogatory act is morally desirable but not required; it is above and beyond the call of duty. One sort of action that is usually thought to be supererogatory is one that involves a great sacrifice on the part of the agent. Thus if one person saved the life of another at the expense of her own life, she would have performed a supererogatory act. Now consider the situation in which carrying the child full term will endanger the life of the woman. The sacrifice that that the woman will have to undergo is very great, so great that it seems implausible to hold that she is morally required to do so. Of course, if she were to sacrifice her own life for that of the child, she would be judged as a very good person. Normally, however, a sacrifice of this magnitude is not morally required of an agent. According to the second approach, then, even if the fetus possesses the right to life, in some circumstances it is permissible to abort it because a woman is not morally required to sacrifice her own life for the well-being of anyone else, including the fetus. This provides the liberal with the same result as the self-defense argument, but for different reasons.

But the second approach does not go far enough; it does not establish anything resembling the liberal position. If it is accepted, one is only committed to the modest proposal that abortion is permissible when carrying the fetus full term will endanger the life or health of the woman. To move beyond this, a *third* approach is needed. The conservative's account of the right to life is mistaken, the liberal argues. To explain the confusion that the liberal attributes to the conservative, let us distinguish between two different interpretations of the right to life. The right to life might be construed as a positive right or a negative right. Consider the interpretation that takes it to be a positive right. If the right to life is a positive right, then others have an obligation to see to it that its possessor has whatever he or she needs to stay alive. On this view, a person has a right to at least the bare minimum necessary to maintain his or her life. By contrast, if the right to life is a negative right, then a person merely has a right against others that they refrain from killing him or her unjustly.[17] On this view, others honor a person's right to life if they refrain from doing certain things; they have no positive duties correlative with this right.

How should the right to life be construed? Is it better understood as a positive right or a negative right? The liberal argues that the right to life must be taken as a negative right, and if it is so understood the conservative's leap from (iii) to (iv) can be seen to be illegitimate. Why must the right to life be interpreted as a negative right? If we take it to be a positive right, absurd results follow. Suppose that a person, $X$, with whom you have no special relationship and to whom you have no special obligations, needs a kidney transplant in order to live. Suppose further that you have two healthy kidneys and are the only person who can serve as a suitable donor for $X$. Are you morally required to donate one of your kidneys to $X$? Surely no one is required to donate a kidney to a perfect stranger, the liberal maintains. Of course, if a person were to do so, it would be a generous act and its agent would be worthy of the highest praise. But to say that such an act is obligatory is much too austere. If the right to life is taken as a positive right, however, it follows that you are morally required to donate your kidney to $X$. After all, according to that view $X$ is entitled to anything necessary for the preservation of life. This shows, then, that the positive interpretation of the right to life is too strong. The right to life is better understood as a negative right.

How does this help the liberal? If the right to life is a negative right, then possessing that right does not guarantee the right to be allowed the continued use of another's body. Of course, if the right to life were a positive right and if having the continued use of another's body were necessary to maintain a person's life, then a person would have this additional right. How this applies to the abortion issue is rather obvious. Even if the fetus possesses the right to life, since that right is negative it does not follow that the fetus possesses a right to the continued use of the woman's body. Since the woman's body is her property, it is reasonable to claim that the fetus has the right to use it only when the woman has given it that right. Unless the woman has given the fetus the right to use her body, then, she may abort it if she wishes.[18] When is it reasonable to say that a woman has given the fetus the right to use her body? There are some clear cases where she has *not* given it this right. If pregnancy has resulted from rape, then certainly the woman has not given the fetus the right to use her body; in such a case she did not even engage in sexual intercourse voluntarily. If the woman has taken all reasonable precautions to avoid pregnancy, if she has used a reliable method of birth control, then it is reasonable to say that she has not given the fetus the right to use her body. However, if the woman engages in sexual intercourse voluntarily, if she uses no means of birth control, if she wants to become pregnant, and if she welcomes the news of her pregnancy, then surely she has given the fetus the right to use her body. There may, of course, be many borderline cases, situations where it is not clear whether the woman has given the fetus the right to use her body. In general, though, if the woman has not voluntarily engaged in sexual intercourse or if she has taken reasonable precautions to avoid pregnancy, then it is plausible to maintain that she has not given the fetus the right to use her body.

Someone might raise the following objection to the third approach just explained. The liberal grants that the fetus possesses the right to life from the moment of conception, but claims that the woman may abort it if she became pregnant because of rape or if she used a generally reliable form of birth control that did not work. But, the objection continues, how can the moral turpitude of the father or the fact that a certain method of birth control did not work affect the fetus's right to life? Why should the father's moral failings weaken the fetus's right to life? The response to this objection is that the fetus's right to life is not weakened; it remains constant throughout. These other factors, however, affect the woman's rights. The fetus's right to life is not the only right at stake; the woman's right to use her body as she wishes is also at stake. And since the right to life is a negative right, the fetus does not automatically possess a right to use another person's body. It has that right only when the other person gives it the right, and when pregnancy results because of rape or the failure of birth control the woman has not given the fetus that right. According to the liberal, then, the fetus's right to life places an obligation on the woman not to abort it only when additional conditions are satisifed.

To summarize this version of the liberal position, recall that the liberal is granting to the conservative that the fetus possesses the right to life from the moment of conception. Contrary to what most have thought, though, it does not follow that abortion is always wrong. The conservative moves much too hastily from the claim that a being possesses the right to life to the assertion that it is always wrong to kill that being. The second and third approaches are designed to establish the liberal position. Let us explain why if these approaches are plausible the liberal position follows. A consequence of the second and third approaches is that abortion is permissible under at least the following conditions: if having the child would be too great a sacrifice or if the woman has not given the fetus the right to use her body. Many are willing to grant that abortion is permissible if the first of these two conditions is satisfied. The second, however, is accepted by far fewer. As long as the woman has taken reasonable precautions to avoid pregnancy, the second reason will allow her to have an abortion for virtually any reason she wants. It is the third approach, then, which makes this position distinctively liberal. It stops short of the radical position, though, because in allowing that the fetus possesses the right to life, it seems to rule out the possibility that infanticide might be permissible.

The key to the version of the liberal position just sketched is the interpretation given to the right to life. If it is granted that the fetus possesses the right to life from the moment of conception and it can still be shown that the liberal position is plausible, this will be a very powerful argument. The plausibility of this position hinges on taking the right to life to be a negative right and on assuming that such a right does not guarantee that its possessor has other rights, such as the right to use another person's body.

At least one apparent oddity of this account of the right to life should be noted. If the claim that an infant possesses the right to life is taken seriously, one would think that this would at least guarantee that the infant also possessed the right to be cared for and nurtured. Without this additional right, the right to life is all but meaningless (for an infant). On its face, it does not seem that the negative interpretation of the right to life can account for this. Of course, if one were to hold that neglecting an infant is just a way of killing it, then the defender of the negative interpretation might argue that the right to be nurtured is a part of the infant's right to life. However, it is hard to see how to avoid extending this to the case of adults too; and then the differences between the positive and negative construals would seem to vanish. In any case, the reader should examine this basic assumption critically and carefully.

### The Moderate Position[19]

The difference between the moderate position and the liberal position is one of degree. The moderate believes that abortion is more difficult to justify than the liberal. Some of the reasons that the liberal provides to justify abortion are regarded by the moderate as unacceptable. It is often claimed that the moderate position is accepted by most people, or at least most people in our society. The decision of the Supreme Court in 1973 reflects the thinking of moderates, at least to some extent. As the name suggests, the moderate attempts to defend a middle-of-the-road position, between the extremes of the conservative and the radical. There are two beliefs which, according to the moderate, are widely shared and which the moderate attempts to incorporate into a position on the abortion issue. The beliefs are these: (1) There is something about the fetus itself, and not merely the social consequences, that makes the practice of abortion morally problematic. (2) Late abortions are more difficult to justify from the moral point of view than early abortions. Most of those on whom the label "moderate" is placed would accept (1) and (2). But how might these two beliefs be justified? Most moderates argue that the fetus becomes a person and so acquires the right to life sometime after conception but before birth. At what point does the fetus become a person? This is the problem of where to draw the line. Moderates have disagreed among themselves about where this point should be. Some have argued that the fetus becomes a person at implantation; others claim that quickening is the crucial point; and still others have urged that viability marks the moment when the fetus obtains the right to life. The problem with any of these approaches is that the growth of the fetus is continuous and it is difficult to see why so much moral weight is put on some specific point in that continuous development. For this reason many have thought that defending the moderate position is hopeless.

Recently, however, a novel defense of the moderate position has been advanced. This new approach combines two approaches more commonly associated with other positions. What this defender of the moderate position wants to do is to account for beliefs (1) and (2) without stipulating at what point the fetus becomes a person and acquires the right to life. To account for belief (1) the moderate will appeal to a weakened version of the potentiality principle. To defend belief (2) the moderate will employ what has been called the conferred claims approach. Let us examine this strategy briefly.

The weakened version of the potentiality principle to which the moderate appeals is this: If, in the normal course of its development, a being will come to have a person's right to life, then by virtue of that fact the being already has some claim to life.[20] This principle tells us, in effect, that a *potential* person has a *claim* to life, while an *actual* person has a *right* to life. A potential person is a being that will become a person in the normal course of its development. Thus a human fetus is a potential person. Neither a human sperm nor an egg is a potential person, though, because neither will become an actual person in the normal course of its development. A right is a rationally demonstrable or valid claim. A person who has a claim is in a position, morally, to demand what is his or her due.[21] Claims, then, including the claim to life, are held with varying degrees of strength; a valid claim must, morally, be honored, while a mere claim need not be. Within this framework a hierarchy of sorts can be established. Some beings have a right to life, for example, adult human beings. Some beings have a claim to life, for example, human beings that are not yet persons. Some creatures, of course, say rats and pigs among others, have neither a right nor a claim to life. If a being has a claim to life, then killing it requires justification. But if a being's claim to life is not as strong as that of an actual person, then such a claim may be defeated by the rights or claims possessed by actual persons. This version of the potentiality principle is weaker than the one attributed to the conservative. The stronger version of this principle gives potential persons the same moral status as actual persons. This weaker version gives potential persons some moral status—in particular, a claim to life—but its moral status is not as great as that of an actual person. Killing a potential person is not a morally neutral act; it requires justification. But it is easier to justify killing a potential person than an actual person.

Why should the weakened version of the potentiality principle be accepted? Certainly it is more plausible than the stronger version. To say that a potential person has the same moral rights as an actual person, as the stronger version does, does not seem correct. Yet potentiality does seem to have some moral force. Humans are regarded as temporal beings, considering their past and their probable future nearly as much as their present. Notice, for example, that as much respect is shown for president-elects and former presidents as is shown for the current president of the United States. And accepting the weakened version of the potentiality principle will explain why there are qualms about experiments performed on human fetuses but no similar reservations concerning experiments done on the fetuses of other animals. If the potentiality principle is plausible, then it provides support for belief (1). All abortions are, to some degree, morally problematic because they involve killing a potential person, and such beings have a claim to life. Thus it is something about the fetus itself—that it is a potential person—that makes abortion an act for which moral justification is required.

But the potentiality principle cannot account for belief (2), that late abortions are more morally problematic than early abortions. Whether a human fetus is one day old or eight months old, it is still a potential person. A different approach is needed to establish the second belief. It should be noted, though, that the potentiality principle that the moderate defends is consistent with belief (2). That is, it is compatible with the potentiality principle that the claims to life held by different people can vary in strength. But why should the claim to life held by a very young human fetus be weaker than the claim to life of an older human fetus? The conferred claims approach is employed at this point by the moderate. The moderate is willing to admit that even a newborn infant does not satisfy all of the necessary and sufficient conditions for personhood. So an infant has only a claim to life. But how strong is this claim? May it be overridden by the mere fact that its parents do not want it? Society may, if it has good reasons for doing so, confer on an infant a very strong claim to life. Even though society must, because of its inherent nature, grant to the fetus some claim to life, it may appeal to other considerations to justify allowing such a claim to vary in strength. And there are good reasons to grant to an infant a much stronger claim to life than is granted to a zygote. The argument supporting such a conferral appeals to the consequences of allowing infanticide and late-stage abortions. Infants are so similar to young persons, the argument goes, that allowing infanticide would create a moral climate in which the right to life of those young persons would be endangered. And by the same reasoning older fetuses are so similar to infants that allowing the former to be killed would endanger the lives of the latter. If society is to protect the right to life of very young persons, then, it has good reasons for conferring on infants and older fetuses a very strong claim to life, a claim so strong that it has the effect of the right to life.

Preventing the implantation of zygotes, however, would surely have virtually no effect on how young persons, infants, or older fetuses are treated. This would suggest, then, that the claim to life of the zygote before implantation is very weak. This approach enables the moderate to avoid the problem of deciding at what point a fetus becomes a person. From conception until sometime after birth the fetus is always a potential person only and so has a mere claim to life; there is no magic moment during pregnancy at which it becomes a person. However, by appealing to the social consequences, society has good reason to allow that claim to life to vary in strength. It is weakest at conception and strongest at birth. And it is natural to hold that its strength increases at certain natural points in the pregnancy, such as implantation, quickening, and viability. At each of these stages, it might be argued, the fetus is becoming more like a person.

Suppose that this latter approach is accepted. What are the consequences for the moral status of abortion and infanticide? It would seem that in the very early stages of pregnancy—certainly before implantation and probably before quickening—abortion for almost any reason is permissible. Certainly the use of IUDs and the prevention of implantation by D. and C. (dilation of the cervix and curettage of the uterus) will be permissible even though they destroy the zygote. Or at least they will be uncontroversially permissible if the woman is too young to be a mother, if the pregnancy is due to rape, or if having the child will be a physical or mental burden. At later stages, though, say after viability, very few reasons will justify abortion. No doubt, if the woman's life or physical health will be endangered by having the child, then abortion will be permissible. The fetus's claim to life is not strong enough to require an actual person to make such a significant sacrifice. But few other reasons will be adequate to override its strong claim to life. And presumably there is no reason that will justify infanticide. Once the child is born, it cannot threaten the well-being of its mother. Of course, the infant's claim to life does not necessarily give it a right against its mother that she care for it. If she is under severe financial strain, it may be that it is society on whom the obligation to care for the child falls. In any case, though, the infant will have such a strong claim to life that it will have the same effect as a person's right to life.

To evaluate this position, two points must be focused on. First, the adequacy of the modified version of the potentiality principle must be determined. The idea behind that principle is to allow the fetus to have some moral status without putting it on a par with adult human beings. Morally speaking, it has a higher status than certain animals, say rats, but a lower status than full-fledged persons. Second, the empirical assertions employed in the application of the conferred claims approach must be examined. Is it really true, for example, that if the lives of older fetuses are taken at will that this will endanger the lives of infants and young persons? It is difficult to determine when an infant becomes a person; as a result, the taking of infants' lives at will might endanger the right to life of young persons. But if, as the moderate admits, infants are not yet persons, then neither are older fetuses. It might then be recommended that we behave as if birth is the point at which a human being becomes a person. One of a liberal persuasion might argue, then, that as long as an infant is never permitted to be killed, killing older fetuses will not endanger the lives of young persons. If this is correct, it is a source of trouble for the moderate in the attempt to establish belief (2). Belief (1) is established, however, if the modified version of the potentiality principle is accepted.

## SUMMARY

One unique feature about the abortion issue is that the extreme views—the conservative and radical positions—often seem more plausible than their competitors. The reason for this might be that most people think that either the fetus possesses the right to life from the moment of conception and therefore abortion is always wrong, or a human being does not come to possess the right to life until after birth and therefore abortion is always permissible. Examining these two extreme views forces a person to focus on the question of what property or properties endow(s) a being with the right to life. Some who defend the conservative view believe that the fetus possesses the right to life from the moment of conception because of genetic endowment or perhaps because God has conferred such a right on all human beings. Radicals reject such an outlook. They argue that properties such as the capacity for self-consciousness are the properties that are morally important. As was seen, however, the conservative can grant the radical this if the conservative can defend the strong version of the potentiality principle. Armed with such a principle, the conservative position can be defended without reverting to genetic endowment or divine conferral as the properties that give a fetus the right to life. It is crucial, then, that this principle be examined carefully.

There is more to the abortion issue than this, however. As was seen in our study of the liberal position, even if it is granted that the fetus possesses the right to life from the moment of conception, it may not follow that abortion is always wrong or even usually wrong. The liberal forces us to ask just what the right to life provides. The liberal presents an interpretation of the right to life, which, if correct, shows that the conservative view on the abortion issue is based on a simple-minded mistake. Finally, the moderate, in effect, grants to the radical that a human being does not obtain the right to life until after birth. But the moderate suggests that to leap from this to the claim that abortion is always permissible is also based on a mistake. A person who makes such a leap is assuming that either a being has a full-fledged right to life or it has no moral status at all. Our conceptual framework is richer than this, though, the moderate suggests. Some beings—in particular, human fetuses—may have a claim to life, although they do not have a right to life. To support this, the moderate appeals to a weakened version of the potentiality principle. If this principle is correct, perhaps a position other than the extreme ones will have some plausibility.

The principal questions concerning the abortion debate, then, are these: What properties are necessary in order for a being to possess the right to life? Does the human fetus, at any stage of its development, possess these properties? Does the fact that a being will come to possess these properties in the natural course of its development give that being either a right to life or a claim to life? And under what conditions is it permissible to kill a being that possesses the right to life?

## CASE STUDY—1

A sixteen-year-old girl is four months pregnant. She became pregnant as the result of rape. Up until this point, the girl had not told anyone about the sexual assault or the pregnancy. She withheld the information because she was afraid. She believes that there is a social stigma attached to victims of rape. She also thinks that her steady boyfriend will reject her if he finds out. And she feels that her parents, who are wealthy socialites, will be ashamed of her and blame her for this predicament. When the girl finally tells her parents what has happened, they decide immediately that she must be taken to another city and have an abortion. The girl agrees, though it is not clear whether she does so because of parental pressure or because she really thinks that it is the best thing to do.

### Discussion Questions

1. Do you think that the parents behaved appropriately in deciding for their daughter that an abortion would be best?
2. Suppose that the physician who is asked to perform the abortion determines that the girl is unsure whether she wants to go through with it. Given that she is already four months pregnant, what should the physician do?
3. Suppose that the girl really does want to have the abortion. How would the conservative evaluate this decision? the radical? the liberal? the moderate?
4. What do *you* think the girl should decide to do?

## CASE STUDY—2

John and Mary have been married for ten years and have three children, all girls. Mary is pregnant again. The couple's income is modest, so having a fourth child will produce a slight but manageable financial strain. However, John and Mary are willing to make sacrifices since they desperately want to have a boy. This has been a dream they have shared since they were married. They realize, of course, that the child might be a girl. When Mary is in her sixteenth week of pregnancy, they learn from a friend about amniocentesis, a procedure in which amniotic fluid surrounding the fetus is withdrawn. The friend tells them that the sex of the child, among other things, can be determined by this procedure. After discussing the matter, John and Mary go to the Prenatal Diagnostic Clinic at the university hospital in their city. When they meet with the physician they tell her that they want to determine the sex of the child that Mary is carrying, and if it is female, Mary will have an abortion.

### Discussion Questions

1. Should the physician agree to perform these tests, given that she knows how John and Mary will use the results? If the physician believes that abortion for sex selection is wrong, should she refuse to do the amniocentesis?
2. Suppose the physician knows that if she does not perform these tests another physician will. How should this influence her decision?
3. Suppose that John and Mary learn that the child is female and decide to abort. How would the conservative evaluate this decision? the radical? the liberal? the moderate?
4. Do you agree with the decision of John and Mary to determine the sex of their unborn child? Explain why or why not.

### SUGGESTIONS FOR FURTHER READING

Baruch A. Brody, "Abortion and the Sanctity of Human Life," in Joel Feinberg (ed.), *The Problem of Abortion* (Belmont, Calif.: Wadsworth Publishing Company, 1973), pp. 104-120.

Daniel Callahan, *Abortion: Law, Choice and Morality* (New York: The Macmillan Company, 1970).

Joel Feinberg, "Abortion," in Tom Reagan (ed.), *Matters of Life and Death* (New York: Random House, 1980), pp. 183-217.

Edward A. Langerak, "Abortion: Listening to the Middle," *The Hastings Center Report*, Vol. 9 (1979), pp. 24-28.

John T. Noonan, Jr., "An Almost Absolute Value in History," in *The Problem of Abortion*, pp. 10-17.

Judith Jarvis Thomson, "A Defense of Abortion," in *The Problem of Abortion*, pp. 121-139.

Michael Tooley, "A Defense of Abortion and Infanticide," in *The Problem of Abortion*, pp. 51-91.

Mary Anne Warren, "On the Moral and Legal Status of Abortion," in Thomas A. Mappes and Jane S. Zembaty (eds.), *Social Ethics* (New York: McGraw-Hill Book Company, 1977), pp. 17-24.

Roger Wertheimer, "Understanding the Abortion Argument," in *The Problem of Abortion*, pp. 33-50.

## NOTES

1. This way of putting the question is suggested by Roger Wertheimer in "Understanding the Abortion Argument," Joel Feinberg (ed.), *The Problem of Abortion* (Belmont, Calif.: Wadsworth Publishing Company, 1973), p. 33.

2. For a discussion of the topic of abortion for the purpose of sex selection, see "Prenatal Diagnosis for Sex Choice," *The Hastings Center Report*, Vol. 10 (1980), pp. 15-20. See also, Holly S. Goldman, "Amniocentesis for Sex Selection," in Marc D. Basson (ed.), *Ethics, Humanism, and Medicine* (New York: Alan R. Liss, Inc., 1980), pp. 81-93.

3. Justice Harry Blackmun, "Majority Opinion in *Roe v. Wade*," in Thomas A. Mappes and Jane S. Zembaty (eds.), *Social Ethics* (New York: McGraw-Hill Book Company, 1977), p. 9. My discussion of the legal status of abortion is limited to the 1973 decisions.

4. Blackmun, "Majority Opinion in *Roe v. Wade*," p. 9.

5. The version of the conservative position that I present here (including most of the criticisms of the other positions) is defended by John T. Noonan, Jr. in "An Almost Absolute Value in History," *The Problem of Abortion*, pp. 10-17. In a few cases I have made changes in the argument so the reader who is interested in Noonan's views should read the article for himself or herself.

6. Of course, those who strictly adhere to Catholic theology hold that it is wrong to practice birth control. They do *not* base their position, however, on the belief that the sperm and the egg have the right to life.

7. In particular, see Noonan, "An Almost Absolute Value in History," pp. 14-15.

8. See Edward A. Langerak, "Abortion: Listening to the Middle," *The Hastings Center Report*, Vol. 9 (1979), p. 26.

9. See Noonan, "An Almost Absolute Value in History," pp. 16-17.

10. This version of the radical position that is presented is argued by Michael Tooley, "A Defense of Abortion and Infanticide," in *The Problem of Abortion*, pp. 51-91. Again, I caution the reader that I have made some changes in the position as I present it. For another paper that seems to be committed to what I call the radical position, see Mary Anne Warren, "On the Moral and Legal Status of Abortion," in *Social Ethics*, pp. 17-24.

11. These are only some of the characteristics suggested by Tooley as ones that are necessary for possession of the right to life. See "A Defense of Abortion and Infanticide," pp. 59-60. For a related but somewhat different account, see Warren, "On the Moral and Legal Status of Abortion," p. 20.

12. Again, though this analysis is taken from Tooley's presentation, his own account is more complex. See "A Defense of Abortion and Infanticide," pp. 60-61.

13. For a more complete discussion of this topic, see Tooley, "A Defense of Abortion and Infanticide," pp. 73-78. The two criteria I discuss here and the criticisms of them are taken from this section.

14. One qualification is needed here. If one's reason for accepting the conservative position is based on religious grounds, then one can argue that there is a morally relevant difference between human fetuses and animal fetuses that does not depend on potential. Such a person might contend that God has endowed human fetuses with the right to life. This is not a position that I shall discuss here. Let us simply note that one who wishes to defend the conservative view on *secular* grounds must accept the potentiality principle.

15. The version of the radical's attack on the potentiality principle presented here is Tooley's and it does depend on the moral symmetry principle. However, Warren presents a different argument against the potentiality principle, one that is not linked to the moral symmetry principle. See her "On the Moral and Legal Status of Abortion," pp. 23-24.

16. The version of what I call the liberal position that I discuss here is presented by Judith Jarvis Thomson, "A Defense of Abortion," in *The Problem of Abortion*, pp. 121-139. I warn the reader again that I have made some changes in the position in my presentation, though they are minor.

17. The qualification "unjustly" is added because the right to life does not give a person the right not to be killed, if, for example, he or she is trying to kill another person.

18. Notice, though, that having the right to abort the fetus is not the same as having the right to kill it. Should the aborted fetus be alive, the woman will not have the right to kill it (assuming that the fetus has the right to life). Of course, the woman will not be required to care for the fetus either.

19. The version of the moderate position that I sketch here is argued for in detail by Edward A. Langerak, "Abortion: Listening to the Middle," pp. 24-28 Again, I have made changes and many omissions, but I have tried to capture the essence of the position.

20. Langerak states this principle differently. Where I use the phrase "a person's right to life" he uses "a person's claim to life." See "Abortion: Listening to the Middle," p. 25.

21. This way of stating the relationship between rights and claims is borrowed from Joel Feinberg, "Rights: Systematic Analysis," in Warren T. Reich (ed.), *Encyclopedia of Bioethics* (New York: The Free Press, 1978), Vol. IV, p. 1508.

# 7

# Social Justice
# and Medicine

Two major topics will be discussed in this chapter. The first deals with the controversies surrounding the right to health care and socialized medicine. Some defend the claim that each person should have equal access to medical care, while others contend that health care must be treated as a good to be sold on the open market. Whether medical workers have the right to strike is the second topic. Some claim that medical workers should never withhold their services; others argue that in certain circumstances medical workers are justified in striking. Each of these issues raises questions about what a just society is and what rights persons have. Thus at the outset the abstract concepts of justice and rights must be explained.

## JUSTICE AND RIGHTS

The term "justice" is used in several different ways in philosophical contexts, and several of these will be distinguished. At the outset, let us distinguish between retributive justice and distributive justice. Questions of retributive justice concern the institution of punishment. When the questions of who should be punished and to what degree are raised, these are matters to which theories of retributive justice address themselves. Other questions of retributive justice include the following: What, if anything, justifies punishing a person? Is capital punishment ever justified? If so, under what conditions? When a mass murderer is convicted, someone might say that this person got his or her just due. When one uses the term "just" in this way, one is referring to retributive justice. These are important questions, but in the context of medical ethics the topic of retributive justice usually does not arise.

Questions of distributive justice deal with how the goods in society ought to be allocated. When one wonders how such goods as food, clothing, shelter, money, political power, and access to health care should be distributed, the issue of distributive justice is raised. To ask whether it is appropriate that some people have more food than they need while others are badly malnourished is to raise a question of distributive justice. Questions of distributive justice arise only when the goods to be allocated are valued by people and relatively scarce. In the past there was never a question about how clean air ought to be allocated since there was an abundant supply of this commodity. Today, however, matters have changed drastically and this now is an issue of distributive justice. Similarly, questions of distributive justice do not arise about grains of sand or handfuls of dirt because normally these are not commodities valued by people. When people ask how health care ought to be distributed in our society or how scarce medical resources ought to be allocated, however, questions of distributive justice are raised. These are commodities that are both valued by people and scarce.

Finally, let us distinguish between formal justice and material justice. The demands of formal justice require that relevantly similar cases be treated in the same way and relevantly different cases in different ways. This notion of justice can be traced back at least as far as Aristotle. What it tells us is that the same criterion must be applied to all cases. It is not appropriate to judge others by one standard and ourselves or our friends by a less rigorous one. One may not make one's own case an exception. The notion of formal justice is, if you will, one step removed from those of retributive justice and distributive justice. Put a different way, whether a question of punishment or one of allocating goods is being considered, the demands of formal justice must be satisfied; in either of these areas, one must treat like cases alike. Merely satisfying the demands of formal justice, however, is not enough. To decide who ought to be punished and how much or to decide how to distribute the goods in our society, one needs to be told more than that one ought to treat like cases alike. That alone provides no guidance. Following only the strictures of formal justice, a person would be unable to say whether another's pay should be determined by his or her need, family size, number of hours worked, the amount of effort exerted, or what. And notice that obviously immoral theories can satisfy the demands of formal justice. A racist theory of distributive justice fulfills the requirements of formal justice in that it applies the same criterion to each case: if you are a member of the preferred race, you will receive favored treatment. And in the area of punitive justice, a theory which requires that the accused prove his or her innocence would pass the test of formal justice if applied to every defendant. Adequate theories of retributive and distributive justice, then, must satisfy the demands of formal justice; but that alone is not sufficient to guarantee their adequacy.

What is lacking in the notion of formal justice is a criterion of relevance. Racist theories of distributive justice are wrong because race is not a relevant factor in determining what goods a person ought to be allocated. That which provides the missing criterion of relevance, whether in the area of retributive justice or distributive justice, is referred to as *material justice*. It might be said, then, that competing theories of distributive justice disagree about what factors are relevant to determining what a person should receive; they disagree on the question of material justice. Later in this chapter two theories of distributive justice will be examined briefly. Proponents of each theory would agree that similar cases should be treated similarly; they disagree, however, on the matter of what factors are relevant to determine what a person should receive.

Let us turn now to the notion of rights. To explain the concept of a right, it is useful to contrast it with that of a privilege.[1] A privilege is a favor bestowed upon someone by a benefactor. It is not something that must be given, nor is it something that can be demanded. If I let someone borrow my copy of *War and Peace*, I am granting a privilege, and this privilege cannot be claimed as one's due. Privileges or favors may be withdrawn by the benefactor at any time. It is appropriate for a person who has been granted a privilege to express gratitude to his or her benefactor. Rights, by contrast, are entitlements that a person possesses. A person's rights give him or her a legitimate claim against others. Rights put restraints on how others may behave toward a person; rights impose obligations on others to act or to refrain from acting in certain ways. And since rights are owed to their possessors, they may not be taken away capriciously. Finally, rights are unlike favors in that it is inappropriate to feel gratitude if one's rights are respected; gratitude is not an appropriate attitude when one has been given what one was owed.

Various kinds of rights can be distinguished. *Moral rights*, let us say, are rights possessed in virtue of one's nature. The moral rights one possesses are not bestowed by society. Instances of moral rights include human rights—the rights possessed in virtue of being a human being—and personal rights—the rights possessed because of being a person. The right not to be killed and the right not to be tortured are two rights often claimed to be both human and personal rights. *Legal rights*, on the other hand, are rights granted by society. On this account, legal rights are conventional. People who live in different countries do not possess the same legal rights. If a person lives in a morally heinous state, many of his or her moral rights will not be recognized as legal rights. For example, in some dictatorial states there is no legal right not to be tortured. Of course, even in a perfectly just state not all of a person's moral rights will also be legal rights. This is because it is inappropriate for the state to enforce all moral rights. Consider this simple example: If a person has saved the life of another at great risk, it is plausible to say that that person has a moral right against the other that he or she express gratitude. But surely no one would advocate making it a law that a benefactor must express gratitude to a good samaritan. Thus even in a perfectly just state not all moral rights will be legal rights.

Other kinds of rights can be distinguished. First, consider the distinction explained previously between negative rights and positive rights. These two differ in the nature of the obligation they impose on others. Negative rights are rights to noninterference. Negative rights impose on others the obligation to refrain from doing certain acts. The right not to be killed is a negative right; others are required to refrain from killing unjustly a person who possesses this right. For the same reasons, the right not to be tortured is negative. Positive rights, on the other hand, are rights to benefits or service. If a person possesses a positive right against a second, the latter is required to perform some particular action or service for the former. If Jones promised Smith that he would help him move, then Smith has a positive right against Jones that he help him move. A second distinction is based on how a person obtains his or her rights. Some rights are possessed *in virtue of one's nature*; in some cases, though, one possesses rights against others only because they have *voluntarily incurred* the correlative obligation. A person's right not to be killed is of the former sort; the right of a promisee against the promisor is of the latter sort. A third distinction is that between *in rem* and *in personam rights. In rem* rights are rights a person holds against everyone or against an entire society. The right not to be tortured is an *in rem* right. If I have the right not to be tortured, every other moral agent is required to refrain from torturing me. Rights that are held against some particular person or persons are called *in personam* rights. The right that a promisee has against the promisor is an *in personam* right; no one but the promisor is obliged to keep the promise. Contracts also give rise to *in personam* rights. The owner of the New York Yankees has an *in personam* right against Reggie Jackson. Having paid him, the owner has a right to Jackson's services on the baseball field.

Typically *in personam* rights are positive and *in rem* rights are negative. If Brown promised Black that she would take care of Black's sick father, then Black has a positive *in personam* right against Brown. Some *in personam* rights, however, are negative rights. If Green's roommate promises her that she will not play her stereo between midnight and dawn, then Green has a negative *in personam* right against her, a right that she refrain from playing the stereo during those hours. Our previous examples, the right not to be killed and the right not to be tortured, are negative *in rem* rights. If a being possesses the right not to be tortured, all moral agents are required to refrain from doing so. Whether there are any positive *in rem* rights is a controversial issue. If an accident victim has a right to be aided by any passerby, then this right is a positive *in rem* one. And if there is a right to health care, it too is a positive *in rem* right. It is positive because it gives one the right to be cared for when one is ill. It is *in rem* because it presumably holds against an entire society. To be sure, medical workers are the persons who administer health care. But it would be ridiculous to say that a person's right to health care was held against a few people simply because they choose to enter a medical profession. If the right to health care is a genuine right, it is similar to a right to be protected against criminals. The latter right is one that is held against one's society, and policemen are persons hired by society to implement and protect this right.

## THEORIES OF DISTRIBUTIVE JUSTICE

Justice is a virtue (and injustice is a vice) that attaches to societies or institutions within society. If there were no organized society—if we had what Thomas Hobbes called "a war of all against all"—the concept of distributive justice would be inapplicable. The notion of distributive justice suggests some sort of intentional distribution of goods, or perhaps a redistribution of goods. The tax structure within any society is an institution which may be graded on the scale of distributive justice. Any tax system clearly involves some sort of redistribution of the wealth. Some have argued that minimum wage laws are necessary in order to fulfill the requirements of distributive justice. And some have supported the welfare system by arguing along these same lines.

Here, two theories of distributive justice will be examined, admittedly at a very superficial level. These views will be called the *liberal* theory of justice and the *conservative* theory of justice. The labels "*the* liberal theory" and "*the* conservative theory" are misnomers because of the many variations on these views.[2] Proponents of these two theories disagree about what constitutes a just society. And it is plausible to say that the source of their disagreement is a dispute about what rights people possess (in a just society). There is some area of agreement between these two theories, though. In Western societies, at least, most would agree about how basic rights should be distributed, such as freedom of movement, political rights, and religious freedoms. These basic rights should be distributed equally. Such basic rights might be called "human goods." Liberals and conservatives alike are egalitarians when it comes to their distribution.

Their disagreement, however, arises concerning the distribution of "economic goods," such as food, clothing, shelter, and money. Put simply, the liberal theory of distributive justice seeks to keep economic and social inequalities at a minimum. It is usually acknowledged that complete economic and social equality is a desirable but not achievable goal. Some jobs are more difficult than others; some are more dangerous than others; some require more time and skill than others. For the good of everyone in our society, good people need to be attracted to these positions. Some incentives must be provided so that intelligent and skilled people will pursue these more difficult jobs. If each person in society were paid the same no matter what position that person held, it is unlikely that many people would seek out the most difficult positions. Therefore in order to benefit everyone in society, persons performing the more difficult tasks must be rewarded accordingly. But how much more should such persons be rewarded? Persons holding these positions should be paid the least amount necessary to encourage the best qualified people to pursue and to keep such jobs.[3] Thus it may be appropriate to pay physicians more than most other people because of the extensive training and long hours required of them. It might also be argued that law enforcement officers should be paid more than most other people because of the dangerous nature of their jobs. Presumably this same line of argument would justify paying the unskilled laborer less than most others make.

The liberal's main point, however, is that these social and economic inequalities must be kept at a minimum. There is an obligation to make the "worst off" people in society as well off as possible. In a real sense society is a joint effort, and its success requires the cooperation of all of its members. If the disparity between the "best off" and the "worst off" in society is too great, the latter will have little or no reason to cooperate. According to the liberal theory, then, people are morally required to structure society so that those at the bottom of the economic ladder are made as well off as possible. This means that the free market must be tampered with. No one may be permitted to charge whatever he or she can get for his or her services. (Or, what amounts to the same thing, if persons are permitted to charge whatever the market will bear, they must be taxed more heavily than those who receive less.) Physicians, for example, will be paid just enough so that the best qualified people will continue to be encouraged to pursue medical professions (a fee that will surely be less than what doctors are making today). If society can be changed in any way so that the "worst off" will be made better off, the "worst off" have a right that such a change be made and all others have an obligation to see to its implementation.

Concerning the distribution of economic goods, conservatives advocate a very different theory of justice. In general, the conservative theory emphasizes individual liberty; in particular, it stresses the importance of property rights. The conservative is opposed to the redistribution of wealth and to taking a person's earnings against his or her wishes except when necessary for the internal or external defense of society. Except for that one special case, however, if a person has acquired his or her wealth legitimately, then the person is entitled to that wealth and no private citizen or government official may seize it. If the wealth is redistributed via taxation to feed the poor, for example, then the persons from whom the money was taken have had their property rights violated.[4] An individual may not be forced to benefit others. No person has a right against others that they render aid to him or her unless those others have voluntarily incurred such an obligation (say, by contracting to do so). Of course, if a person chooses to help another, he or she may do so. But this is an act of charity or a supererogatory act, not a moral requirement.

Notice that if the worst off in a society possess a right to be made as well off as possible, as the liberal maintains, this is a positive *in rem* right. It is positive because it is a right to receive goods from others (directly or indirectly); it is *in rem* because it holds against an entire society. Liberals, then, unlike conservatives, are committed to the claim that there are positive *in rem* rights. If there are positive *in rem* rights, then it follows that there are natural duties; that is, duties to aid others that a person has merely because he or she is a moral agent and not because that person voluntarily incurred such duties. Again, the liberal finds this consequence acceptable, but the conservative does not. Finally, the liberal maintains that there is an obligation to bring about a distribution of economic goods as equal as possible. The conservative disagrees. According to the conservative, as long as no one cheats, defrauds, or steals from another, each person is entitled to whatever he or she earns and no one has a right to take it. If a nearly equal distribution arises when the market is allowed to be free, that is quite appropriate; if a grossly unequal distribution arises, that is fine too. This, then, is a very brief look at the liberal and conservative theories of distributive justice.

## THE RIGHT TO HEALTH CARE

Today it is frequently said that there is a health care crisis in the United States. Never before has the health care system been subjected to more criticism. Yet in some respects this is puzzling.[5] Today there are more people working in medical professions than ever before. There are more than enough hospital beds in the United States. On any given day, there are thousands of empty beds in hospitals. More people than ever have some sort of medical insurance to cover the cost of their health care. This is because of the advent of Medicare and Medicaid, and because many businesses now extend to their employees some sort of health insurance. More money is being spent on health care than ever before. And this is not merely due to inflation; over the past few decades a greater percentage of the Gross National Product has been poured into the delivery of health care. When one adds to this the many advances made in medicine over the last few years and that more illnesses can be cured than ever before, one may wonder why anyone would say that there is such a crisis.

In spite of the many successes, however, there are problems with the health care system in the United States. First, though there are more medical workers than ever before, the number of physicians, nurses, and other medical personnel is still too small in certain areas of the country. In particular, in inner-city ghettos and rural areas there are too few doctors and nurses. But in the wealthy suburbs there are more than enough medical workers. Second, the delivery of health care in the inner-city ghettos and in rural America is inadequate. This is, in part, due to the shortage of medical workers; the lack of adequate facilities and equipment is also a contributing cause. Third, there is a great inequality in our health care system. Those from middle and upper classes seem to get much better health care than the poor, especially poor blacks.[6] Finally, health care costs are rising at a meteoric rate, a rate much faster than other items in our economy. It is these factors (and some others), then, that have led many to be critical of the health care system in our country today. The problem rests in the distribution of health care. The scientific and technological advances that have been made are very impressive. But many feel that these are not being allocated fairly. The critics charge that even with these advances too many people are receiving inadequate health care.

It is in this climate that the slogan "the right to health care" was born. What does it mean to say that people have the right to health care? As was stated earlier, if health care is a right, then surely it is a positive *in rem* right.[7] Minimally, to say that people have a right to health care is to say that all people ought to have access to health care independent of their financial means or social status. And in this context "right" means a morally justified claim. If there is a right to health care, then, each person is entitled to such care. It should be realized, however, that this is a right that can only be recognized in a relatively wealthy society. It would not be plausible to say that persons in a poor, overpopulated country had a right to health, since the correlative obligation that society would have to provide for health care would be impossible to fulfill. Do the citizens of a relatively wealthy country have a right to health care? It can be argued quite credibly that it is in the interest of society to provide adequate health care for its people. This is so because everyone benefits from the prevention of medical catastrophes: a society is crippled when hit with a plague or an epidemic. Moreover, society benefits if each of its members is a working, productive citizen. But to say that society has an interest in providing health care for its citizens is not the same as saying that those persons have a right to such care. All this shows is that there is a consequentialist argument which suggests that society will be better off if it provides minimally acceptable health care for its members. But if citizens have a right to health care, they have a claim against society to provide it regardless of whether it benefits the society as a whole.

## HEALTH CARE AS A RIGHT: THE COMPETING VIEWS

If one has a right to health care, it is a right against one's society. And it seems clear that the only way society can provide health care for all of its citizens is through revenue acquired from taxes. Thus if a society actually provides people with health care, some redistribution of wealth will be required. Should a society that can do so pay, fully, or in part, for the health care of its members? What will be called the *conservative* view on this issue is simple: the answer to this last question is no. Health care is not something to which a person has a right; rather it is something which may be purchased. As the conservative sees it, health care is a service provided by doctors, nurses, and other medical workers which is sold on the market to anyone who can afford it and who wishes to buy it. Just like automobiles and pastries, health care is a commodity the price of which should be determined by the free market. How the conservative recommends handling certain problems within the health care professions is a topic to which we shall return later.

By contrast, the *liberal* argues that health care is a basic right, at least for persons in a relatively wealthy society. A just society will provide the apparatus to insure that each of its citizens has the opportunity to receive adequate health care. Health care is (or should be) just as much a right as life, liberty, and the pursuit of happiness. According to the liberal, a society which permits the wealthy to receive excellent health care and the poor to receive little or no health care is unjust. Since it is the liberal who claims that society has a positive obligation to provide health care for its citizens, let us see one way in which this view might be defended.

## THE LIBERAL VIEW

As was seen earlier, the claim that there is a crisis in our health care system today is based partly on the fact that a person's income and geographic location greatly affects the quality of medical care received. The liberal will argue that each person should receive health services regardless of financial or geographical considerations. The strategy employed by the liberal is to consider different criteria that might be used for distributing health care and to argue that all but the liberal criterion are inadequate.[8] The first criterion to be examined is this: To each according to his or her own merit. According to this criterion, goods should be distributed in accordance with the worth or merit of those competing for the goods. This criterion, however, requires further explanation. There are two different senses in which a person might be said to merit or deserve something. On the one hand, a person might deserve something because of his or her objective achievements; here merit is related to the actual results of a person's acts. On the other hand, it might be said that a person deserves something because of the effort exerted or because of what that person was trying to do, regardless of the actual results produced. It seems plausible to maintain that some goods or rewards should be distributed in accordance with a person's objective achievements. The Nobel prize in chemistry, for example, should surely be given to the person who made the most outstanding contribution or discovery in the field of chemistry, irrespective of the effort put forth or the hours of work spent. Similarly, the grade a student receives should be determined by his or her objective achievements. In other contexts, though, it has been suggested that goods or rewards should be allocated according to a person's efforts or motives. Some people who, for religious reasons, believe in life after bodily death hold that entrance into heaven depends on efforts and the goodness of one's motives, not on actual achievements. And our legal system takes into account a person's motives and intentions. The person who meticulously planned a murder is punished more severely than the person who kills another in a moment of passion.

However appropriate either version of this first criterion might be in some situations, though, the liberal rejects it as a basis for distributing health care. The principal reason for rejecting this criterion is that there is a lack of fit between merit and the reason health crises occur. That is, illnesses often occur for reasons that are beyond a person's control. Diseases afflict the saint and the sinner indiscriminately. In contexts where it is appropriate to use merit or desert as the basis for distributing goods, luck plays less of a role. The potentially brilliant student who fails because of laziness deserves his or her grade. But it is not normally said that a person deserves to be ill. Therefore it would be inappropriate to distribute health care according to merit. It might be said, of course, that in some cases a person is responsible for his or her illness. A heavy cigarette smoker who contracts lung cancer might be said to be responsible for that illness. And a person who is seriously injured in an autombile accident caused by driving while drunk might be said to have brought about any injuries resulting from that accident. So, the critic might argue, in some cases merit is related to illness and health care should be allocated accordingly. The liberal responds to this, though, by pointing out the great number of practical problems this would involve. Should we say that a football player who receives a serious head injury is responsible for his own condition? Is an obese person who has a heart attack responsible for her condition? Clearly physicians, nurses, and other medical workers are not in a position to make such judgments, and so allocating health care according to merit will not work for practical reasons. It may be appropriate, though, to raise the taxes on cigarettes and use the additional funds to cover the extra cost imposed on the health care system by the smoker. In this way people might be forced to pay for the illnesses that are, in effect, self-inflicted.

A second criterion that might be put forth as the basis for distributing health care is this: To each according to his or her social contributions. This criterion appeals to the notion of utility. It suggests that health resources be allocated to those who are most useful to society. This criterion may be appropriate in allocating some goods. It may, for example, be an appropriate basis for determining a worker's salary. Certainly many think that it is because of the nature of their contributions to society that we are justified in paying physicians more than janitors and petroleum engineers more than teachers. But should health care be distributed on the same basis? In treating illnesses, should priority be given to those who make greater societal contributions? The liberal argues that it should not. Several reasons are offered to support this contention. First, there again seems to be a lack of fit between societal contributions and the reason health crises occur. In fact, through no fault of their own, those with serious diseases who need health care the most are the persons least able to contribute to society. Among others, this would include the aged, the disabled, and children. If this were the criterion used to distribute health care, those who need it the least would be given top priority and those who need it the most would be last in line. There seems to be something untoward about this. Second, to distribute something as necessary as health care on the basis of societal contributions seems to conflict with our belief that people are equal. Using this criterion suggests that the greater a person's societal contribution is, the more worthy that person is. Finally, the idea that a person's societal usefulness can be estimated seems doubtful. Men as great as Socrates and Thoreau were considered to be societal menaces by their contemporaries. For these reasons, then, the second criterion does not seem appropriate for allocating health care.

The third criterion of distributive justice to be considered is the following: To each according to his or her ability to pay.[9] This is the conservative view. The medical worker is one who has a service to sell. Such a view, the conservative argues, honors the free choices of people. The medical worker, the baker, and the entertainer are all private entrepreneurs. They may charge whatever they wish for their services. If their prices are unreasonable, people will not buy the service and this, plus competition, will force the price down. If a company is willing to pay a television actor millions of dollars a year, either it is profitable for it to do so or it believes that it is in its best interests. In either case, it is their free choice. This same law of supply and demand should be permitted to operate in the medical profession. If a physician is charging too much, competitors will drive that physician out of business. If a patient believes that all physicians charge too much for a certain service, that patient need not buy it.

To this view the liberal has two major objections. First, it is very misleading to compare medical workers, especially physicians, with other private entrepreneurs. The analogy is a false one. The physician cannot claim to be independent in the same way that the baker, the entertainer, or the professional football player can. The physician (and other medical workers) is dependent on others and to a large degree has already incurred a debt to society (in a way that the baker and entertainer have not). This is so because physicians cannot even do their work without the support and cooperation of hospitals, nurses, medical technicians, and nonmedical personnel employed by the hospital. Moreover, the medical worker has a debt to the public because much of the money that is given to support medical research is supplied by the taxpayer and taxpayers contribute greatly to the education of medical workers. The second objection to the conservative view is that it is inappropriate to regard medical care as an item on the free market which one need not buy. When medical catastrophes strike, all people must seek the services of a physician. Unlike the baker and the entertainer, the medical worker is supplying a service that the consumer must purchase.

The fourth criterion, and the one favored by the liberal, is this: To each according to his or her needs. Since health care is a necessity and since medical crises strike people indiscriminately and unpredictably, a society that can afford to do so will be unjust unless it supplies health care to its citizens according to need. The intention, though, is that only basic health care needs will be provided by society. Optional treatment must be paid for by the patient. Drawing a precise line between basic treatment and optional care may be difficult, but there are clear cases of each. Treating pneumonia or breast cancer is fulfilling a basic need; plastic surgery normally is not. If this criterion is accepted, then each person's basic medical needs must be paid for with public monies. But why should this view be accepted? A just society, it might be argued, must provide its citizens with at least their essential needs. A person should gain something by being a member of society. If a person does not gain something, then he or she has no motive for obeying society's laws. And if society ought to provide its citizens with anything, surely it should tend to their essential needs first. Food, clothing, shelter, fuel, and health care are all essential needs. And it can be argued that even among these indisputable essentials, health care is special. People can prepare for emergencies in the other areas in a way that they cannot prepare for medical crises. Food can be preserved and fuel can be stored in anticipation of shortages, but there is nothing a person can do to prepare for a medical crisis. Moreover, medical catastrophes seem to be very unpredictable. People are more vulnerable to crises in this area than in any of the others. So if a just society should insure that its citizens' essential needs are met, it certainly should guarantee that they receive basic health care.

If the fourth criterion is convincing, one might think that that is the end of the story. But at least some liberals think that it is not.[10] A fifth criterion is needed: Similar treatment for similar cases. This is an appeal to what was earlier called formal justice. But why is this additional criterion necessary? The fourth criterion, the need-conception of justice, implies that it would be wrong to allow one person to receive better health care than another because of factors such as income and geographic location. What the fourth criterion requires is that each person have equal access to health care as needed. But not all societies are affluent enough to provide for all of their citizens' basic needs. In these less-than-optimal circumstances, how should medical care be distributed? It is at this point that the fifth criterion is needed. Even in less-than-optimal circumstances, wealth or geography should not determine who receives health care. Rather similar treatment should be provided for similar cases. In these unfortunate situations health care should be allocated according to categories of illness. For example, all other things being equal, it would be a reasonable policy to treat persons with a communicable disease before treating those with a noncommunicable disease. And it would be a sensible policy to give priority to those who have a common illness that is easily treated ahead of those who have a rare disease the treatment of which is costly and uncertain. The point is that impartial criteria must be employed to determine who receives health care when not all can.

The principal idea underlying the liberal view can be shown by the following example. Suppose that there are two different children each of whom has the same rare disease. One is from a very wealthy family and the other is from a very poor family. Unless health care is a right that each person has, these two children will receive very different care. The one from the very wealthy family will receive the best care available and the one from the poor family will get little or no medical attention. Yet this seems unfair. Each child has the same need and neither can be said to deserve his or her fate. One is lucky enough to have parents who can afford the best medical care; the other is not. But surely, if it can be prevented, luck should not play a role in a matter of life or death. By citing the case of the children, then, liberals hope to convince others that need should be the sole determinant of who receives health care. Certainly the income of one's parents or where one's parents happen to live should not be influential factors.

## IMPLEMENTING THE LIBERAL VIEW

If health care is a right, as the liberal urges, then society must set up the machinery to provide it for its citizens. How this might be done is a difficult problem for policy makers. Two different programs shall be sketched which might be used in order to make health care equally accessible to all people.[11] The first of these programs is a classical form of third-party payments, usually called National Health Insurance. This is a system in which the government pays the medical worker for delivering basic health care services to the patient. Details of such a program will vary from proposal to proposal. Some may require a citizen to pay for a certain amount of health care—until the costs exceed a percentage of his or her taxable income—and then have the government pay any additional costs. Some may not pay for those whose incomes are very great—say, in excess of $50,000 per year. What is common to each, though, is that medical workers remain private entrepreneurs. Physicians, for example, are still in practice for themselves and set their own prices. They are paid, however, in part or in full, by the government rather than the patient. This system, in effect, guarantees that medical workers will be paid for their services. And the system still allows a person to purchase his or her own health care if that is the person's preference. It also allows for the purchase of additional medical treatment beyond what the government will pay for. That the system allows these things is evidence of what its major purposes are. It is not designed to insure that each citizen will receive equal health care. Its paramount purpose is to guarantee that each person will have his or her fundamental health care needs fulfilled adequately. It is also designed to protect people from medical catastrophes; that is, its intent is to insure that no one will be placed in dire financial straits because of a medical problem.

A somewhat different program is one that involves a complete federalization of the health care system. Such a program is sometimes called National Health Service or socialized medicine. In this system medical workers are not private entrepreneurs; rather they are employed by the government and are presumably paid on a salaried basis. The purpose of this system is more radical than that of National Health Insurance: its aim is to guarantee that each person receives equally adequate health care, namely, the best health care available for that person's particular medical problems. No one should gain an advantage because of his or her wealth. Nor is anyone significantly disadvantaged because of his or her geographic location. In such a system, not only does the government handle the financing of all medical care, but it also controls the entire health care structure. It will determine the salary of medical workers, assign them their place of work, and even control admission to medical schools and schools of nursing. If it is to insure that neither geography nor lack of wealth will adversely affect a person's chances of receiving quality medical care, then it must have this sort of control. The health care system is supported solely by tax monies. As a citizen and presumably a taxpayer or a dependent of one, a person is entitled to seek health care whenever he or she believes that it is necessary. Since medical workers will be assigned to work in various areas, this insures, to the degree that it is possible to do so, that each person will have trained medical personnel within a reasonable commuting distance.

## OBJECTIONS TO THE LIBERAL VIEW

Conservatives often defend their own position by pointing out difficulties with systems involving third-party payments and socialized medicine. In general, conservatives claim that no matter how the liberal ideal is enacted, it will involve a loss of liberty for that nation's citizens. But more specific criticisms are raised, some of which will be discussed here.

First, the conservative charges that neither a system of third-party payments nor national health service will guarantee an improvement in the quality of health care. The immediate beneficiaries, at least in a system of third-party payments, will be the medical profession itself. What such a system does is to insure that medical workers will be paid for the services they render.

Second, if the state gains even partial control of the health care system, many individual rights will be placed in jeopardy or denied. In particular, two very important rights will be threatened: the right of the patient to refuse treatment and the right of the physician to refuse to treat a patient. To explain these claims, consider again the case of the 57-year-old woman with cancer of the cervix (discussed in Chapter Three). Suppose that she refuses treatment and will not change her mind. What is likely to happen? The woman's condition will get progressively worse. She will occupy the hospital bed for a longer time, she will require much more attention from physicians and nurses than she would have had she had the hysterectomy, and as a result the cost of her health care will be much greater. But if the state is paying for her treatment, it cannot allow her to burden the system in this way. The state has a legitimate interest in keeping the cost of health care down, and in order to achieve this end it must sometimes force treatment on patients against their will. Imagine the enormous drain on the health care system if a patient refused treatment and as a result lapsed into a long-term, irreversible coma. Physicians will not be permitted to refuse to treat a patient either. If health care is a right that citizens have against their society, then medical workers are simply instruments of society for carrying out this right. Medical workers would be in a position similar to that of policemen. Clearly an officer of the law may not refuse to protect a citizen when his or her rights are being threatened. Similarly, if health care is a right a citizen possesses, then doctors and nurses will not be permitted to refuse to treat a patient with a legitimate medical need. Thus a Roman Catholic obstetrician may be forced to perform an abortion even though he or she has moral and religious objections to such a procedure.[12]

The third objection raised by conservatives is that a system in which health care is paid for by the state will jeopardize the confidentiality of the medical worker-patient relationship. As was seen earlier (in Chapter Two), it is very important for patients to be able to communicate freely with medical workers, and they will do so only if they believe that such communications remain confidential. But if health care is paid for from public monies, then there must be checks built into the system to minimize abuse. Included among these checks will be the requirement that physicians fill out reports detailing the treatment administered to the patient in question. After all, if a physician is to be paid, the government must be sure that some service was actually rendered. Thus the state has a legitimate interest in knowing what sort of treatment a patient received. That medical workers will be forced to make such reports, however, will have a serious effect on their relationship with the patient. The patient will be more inclined to withhold potentially embarrassing information. The patient may even come to regard the medical worker as an adversary or an agent of the state.[13] So not only will the right of confidentiality be jeopardized, but the medical worker-patient relationship will be threatened too.

The fourth objection is by far the most common one. When the major portion of medical costs is borne by someone other than the patient, as it will be if the liberal view is enacted, then the possibilities of abusing the system are almost unlimited. To confirm this, note the many scandals associated with the Medicare and Medicaid programs in the United States over the last few years. Both the patient and the medical worker can abuse systems of this sort. The effect of these abuses is that medical costs will soar. But what are some of the more specific abuses that are likely to occur?

First, it is likely that the demand for health care will increase dramatically. If someone else is paying for medical treatment, people will go to the doctor for every little ache or pain. This is human nature, the critic claims. If a person is traveling on the company's expense account, he or she will go first class; but if it is the traveler who is paying the bill, corners will be cut and luxuries will be foregone. If this view of human nature is correct, then a likely consequence of making health care a right is that doctors' offices will be overcrowded and a bed in a hospital will be hard to find. Next, medical workers will be tempted to abuse the system too. If a form of National Health Insurance is adopted and physicians remain private entrepreneurs, they may be tempted to file false reports—to submit more charges and services that they actually performed. Moreover, many doctors will be tempted to see as many patients as they can since it will be lucrative for them to do so. This latter problem has already surfaced since the implementation of Medicare and Medicaid. On the other hand, if a form of National Health Service is adopted, making medical workers salaried employees, they might become lax. Since it would not affect their pay, physicians would be tempted to see as few patients as possible. And their attitudes toward patients are apt to be more impersonal. Finally, if the government takes over the entire medical structure, hospital administrators will try to purchase all of the exotic medical machinery and technology that they can. And patients, in turn, will be inclined to opt for more expensive and elaborate treatment than they would otherwise seek.

The conservative's fifth objection applies to any version of the state's paying for the medical costs of its citizens. If this happens, it is argued, the total cost of medical care will increase without any attendant increase in the quality of health care. If the government pays for health care, a new bureaucracy will have to be created, namely, those persons who monitor the system, check for abuses, make payments, and the like. What is worse is that these new employees provide no medical service to the patients. They are middlemen, if you will, who contribute nothing to health care as such. It seems unwarranted to allow the costs of medical care to increase in this way.

The final objection to be considered here is a more general one. If the state becomes the supplier of medical care, many serious and difficult questions concerning matters of public policy will arise that can be avoided if medicine remains in the private sphere. For example, policymakers will have to determine what is considered a genuine illness or disease. Is ordinary obesity, due to eating too much, a disease that ought to be treated? Is being pregnant when that is undesirable (and there are no other medical complications) an illness? Is a hair transplant or plastic surgery legitimate medical treatment for which the state ought to pay? Even more troublesome is the ill person who might be responsible for his or her own condition. Should the state pay for that person's treatment? For example, if a heavy smoker contracts lung cancer, should society pay for that person's medical care? And if a person works at a dangerous occupation, say that of a coal miner, must society bear the additional costs of medical care if that person comes down with black lung disease?[14] These are but a few of many difficult questions that must be answered if the liberal view is to be implemented. Other problems arise too. If health care is placed entirely in the hands of the government, steps will be taken to make it as efficient and economical as possible. Certainly one thing which will contribute to this end is an aggressive program of preventive medicine. But how aggressive may this program be? If each person received a complete physical examination annually, there is no doubt that many potentially serious medical problems would be detected early and prevented. In the long run this would probably lead to better and less costly medical care. If the state is paying for all of our health care, will it have a right to compel us to undergo annual physical examinations? And perhaps the state will have to consider seriously offering financial incentives to those who practice good preventive medicine through a program of vigorous exercise, such as bicycling, running, or swimming. That all of these hopelessly complex questions even arise shows the problems involved with socialized medicine, the conservative contends.

## THE CONSERVATIVE VIEW: SOME FINAL THOUGHTS

The conservative believes that if health care remains a good on the free market to be purchased if one chooses, there will be certain advantages. For one thing, certain rights that we cherish, such as the right of confidential communications with medical workers, the right to refuse treatment, and the right of the medical worker to refuse to treat a patient, will be protected. Moreover, when health care is treated as a good to be purchased, both patients and medical workers are provided with incentives to keep medical costs at a minimum. Since patients are paying for their own health care, they will go to a physician only when it is necessary and they will demand exotic, expensive treatment only as a last resort. Physicians, on the other hand, will be motivated to provide high quality care since they will want the patient to return and to tell others about their service. And if the market is truly free, prices will remain at a reasonable level because of competition. Finally, if society adopts the conservative position, we need not worry about such questions as what constitutes a genuine illness. Since it is the patient who is paying for medical care, he or she may act as the sole arbiter concerning what conditions should be treated and which should not.

Some have accused the conservative of being a callous, morally insensitive person. Surely neither the conservative nor anyone else can deny that there are serious problems in our health care system today. Geography and wealth do play signficant roles in determining the quality of health care that a person receives. And even the conservative must admit the medical costs are inordinately high today and escalating at a rate faster than general inflation. What, then, does the conservative say about these problems? Must society simply live with them, or does the conservative offer some relief?

The conservative maintains that if the market is free, then most of the problems associated with the delivery of health care will disappear. Consider the lack of physicians in rural areas. The solution to this problem is already emerging through the operation of the free market. Today many rural communities are making contracts with medical students. Members of the community raise enough money in order to pay the student's way through medical school, and in exchange he or she agrees to serve for a certain number of years in that community. Such arrangements are becoming commonplace today, and this is certainly a step in the right direction with regard to solving this problem. What does the conservative say about the exorbitant cost of medical care today? Costs are too great today because a seller's market has been created. The demand for physicians is much greater than the supply. However, the conservative contends, such a market has been artificially created. In particular, the AMA has been able to keep the supply of physicians sufficiently low to protect their own financial interests. Because of their control of the accreditation of medical schools and because of their influences over licensure boards, they have subtly but effectively insured that the supply of doctors will not get too great.[15] Finally, since any form of state intervention in the health care system is opposed, what does the conservative propose to do about the plight of the elderly who have retired but whose medical costs have increased? In a free market it will be profitable for insurance companies to develop policies which will handle the health care costs of a person after he or she has retired. It will be rational for each person to buy such a policy in order to protect future interests. The companies will make their profit from the premiums of all of those who never need to file a claim (either because of an early death or because of excellent health). The costs of such policies will be reasonable because if a company is charging too much, another will offer a less expensive policy in order to lure customers to it. Of course, some people may not buy such policies. What happens to them if they become ill? A consistent conservative will presumably say that unless there are friends, relatives, or altruistic strangers who are willing to pay for their care, they will have to go without. Conservatives might hope that in a country such as ours charitable organizations will arise to handle such problems. If this were not to occur, however, the imprudent would have to go without health care.

The problems underlying the liberal view on the right to health care are serious. In addition to the points already discussed, many object that implementation of the liberal program involves forcing some persons to benefit others. It is compulsory good samaritanism, if you will. Whether free market principles are the panacea for all of the problems surrounding the delivery of health care, as the conservative believes, however, is a matter for further debate.

## UNIONIZATION AND THE RIGHT TO STRIKE FOR MEDICAL WORKERS

Do medical workers have the right to unionize and to strike? At the outset, the context in which this question is raised should be explained. With only a minor qualification to be added later, it can accurately be said that issues of unionization and striking do not arise as long as medical workers are private entrepreneurs. A physician who is not satisifed with his or her salary may raise prices. And any doctor who is unhappy with the required work hours may cut back on the number of patients he or she is seeing. If, however, the government becomes involved in the health care system, then the medical worker is directly or indirectly an employee of the state. The medical worker will have lost some independence and autonomy. To avoid becoming "pawns" in the hands of the state, medical workers must consider seriously the possibility of forming unions and, if necessary, withholding their services. If one cannot control one's working conditions and if one is dissatisfied with aspects of those conditions, then one will be tempted to unionize and to consider seriously the possibility of striking.

Physicians and nurses have engaged in strikes and work slowdowns. It is customary, though, that during such periods emergency services are still provided. What is withheld are "routine" medical services. In 1975 and 1976 doctors in California and New York engaged in slowdowns.[16] Residents and interns in New York, Chicago, and Los Angeles went on strike during this same period. And physicians in Saskatchewan, Quebec, and Chile engaged in mass strikes during the 1960's and 1970's. Let us examine some of the reasons that were given by the participants in these slowdowns and strikes to justify their actions.

First, the slowdowns staged by the California and New York physicians were prompted by drastic premium hikes in malpractice insurance. Their aim was to exert pressure on their state legislatures to take action to prevent these increases. A second reason that has been given to justify the withholding of services concerns the number of hours that medical workers must put in. Among the demands made by the residents and interns who struck was that the number of hours worked per week, which often exceeded 100 hours, be reduced to 80. They claimed, quite plausibly, that a person who put in a 120-hour work week could not serve his or her patients adequately. The demand that patient-care facilities be improved is a third reason sometimes given to justify strikes by medical workers. Because a significant number of their patients spoke only Spanish, one of the demands of the Chicago interns and residents was for Spanish translators. They reasoned, quite plausibly, that if they spoke only English and their patients spoke only Spanish, the chances that they could provide adequate patient-care were not good. In 1976 nurses at Cook County Hospital went on strike. Their chief demand was also related to the quality of patient-care: they wanted the critical care units to be more fully staffed.[17] The fourth reason that might be given to justify withholding medical services, and the one that was actually given by doctors in Saskatchewan, Quebec, and Chile, is this: to prevent the government from implementing some form of national health insurance. As was seen earlier, physicians argue that not only will a government takeover of the health care system affect their financial status, but it also constitutes an intrusion on the doctor-patient relationship. Striking is a means designed to prevent what is regarded as an undesirable end. A fifth reason that might be given to justify a strike by medical workers is to obtain a salary increase. As things stand now, others are not likely to think of this as a reason for justifying a strike by physicians. They are, after all, being paid quite well. For many other medical workers, however, this may be a very plausible reason for withholding their services. Consider, for example, the situation of nurses. It was reported in 1978 that the average salary range for nurses was between $14,000 and $17,500 per year.[18] When one realizes that plumbers and brewery workers, to cite but two examples, make more than this, it can be seen more clearly why financial considerations may provide a good reason for withholding medical services. And if doctors were to become salaried employees of the state, this reason may justify their withholding services too.

Let us now investigate the connection between collective bargaining and a just distribution of social goods.[19] The power of collective bargaining provides an opportunity to press claims against others. But the mere fact that there is such an opportunity does not insure that a just result will ensue. Unless one believes that any outcome of bargaining on the free market is necessarily just, it must be admitted that some outcomes may be unfair. Winning through collective bargaining is a matter of strength. If management has labor at a disadvantage, then it is likely that the former will win in the process of the collective bargaining. Certainly in the early days of the union movement this is exactly what happened. When the situations are reversed, labor will win most of its demands. None of this is to deny the importance of having the opportunity to press one's claims against others. Nor is it to deny that unionization has provided many with the chance to gain what seems to be a fair salary. The point is simply that the process of collective bargaining may not always produce results that seem to be fair.

## ARGUMENTS AGAINST UNIONIZATION AND THE RIGHT TO STRIKE

There are many who believe that medical workers should never unionize or threaten to withhold their services. Several arguments might be given to support this position. One argument rests on the claim that there is a conflict between the professionalism that medical workers should exhibit and the idea of unionization. The argument can be sketched as follows.[20]

1. Physicians, nurses, and other medical workers are professionals, and professionals have certain special obligations, such as a commitment to enhancing the standards of their profession, holding their colleagues to high standards of performance, and the like.
2. Physicians and nurses have a special professional relationship with patients, a relationship that places special obligations on them to provide patients with the best care they can, to cultivate trust, to maintain confidentiality, and the like.
3. This professional relationship will be threatened or damaged if patients believe that doctors and nurses are motivated significantly by monetary concerns rather than professional duty.

4. Unions are perceived by the general public primarily as instruments for advancing the self-interest of their members.
5. Therefore if physicians or nurses have unions or even the possibility of striking, patients will believe that they are motivated primarily by monetary concerns and this will mean that the medical worker will be unable to fulfill his or her special obligations (such as cultivating trust).

Let us assess this argument. The first two premises seem to be plausible. In asserting that professionals have special obligations to their clients, one is simply saying that the role one plays can generate new obligations. The numerous codes of ethics for the various professions suggest that this is a widely shared belief. That the professional obligations of medical workers include the maintenance of trust and confidentiality is neither a controversial nor novel idea. But what about the third premise? The claim here seems doubtful. Anyone who asserts this premise must think that patients are very naive. Patients are depicted as persons who believe that medical workers are motivated solely by altruistic considerations. If they find out that medical workers are concerned about financial matters too, they will lose their trust and confidence in those workers. Surely, though, patients are not this naive. Surely most patients believe that medical workers are motivated by several considerations, two of which are the desire to help and the desire to enhance their financial status. If medical workers care about the health of their patients, the presence of additional considerations will not cause the patient to lose confidence in the worker. Of course, if patients believed that medical workers were concerned *only* about financial matters, this would undermine the relationship. What the patient is most concerned about is the attitude of the medical worker, and a medical worker who is motivated only by the desire to make money is not likely to express any concern for the welfare of the patient. The third premise, then, is false.

But is the fourth premise true? It is probably accurate to say that most people do regard unions as instruments for advancing the interests of their members. However, if such a perception is mistaken, it can be corrected. Many who have argued that medical workers should unionize believe that unions can advance the interests of both the workers and the patients. Unions can, for example, work for the improvement of patient-care facilities. The case of the residents of Cook County Hospital demanding Spanish translators is an excellent example of how unions might press for the interests of patients too. To insure that the relationship with the patient is not undermined, however, medical workers have a derived obligation to explain the dual function that unions can play. That is, they must make sure that the public does not misunderstand the goals of the union. They must make patients aware that the union is fighting for their interests as well as those of the medical workers. Given that this sort of public education can take place, the plausibility of premise four can be called into question. This first argument, then, is not very convincing.

A second argument, and undoubtedly the one most commonly accepted, that medical workers should neither unionize nor strike appeals to the nature of the risks involved if medical services are withheld. The argument can be sketched as follows.

1.  If medical workers are allowed to withhold their services, the risks will be great. In particular, the health of many people will be affected adversely, and some may even die.
2.  But medical workers should never take actions that seriously threaten the health of their patients or of innocent persons. This is contrary to their professional obligations.
3.  Therefore medical workers should never withhold their services from their patients or from other innocent parties.[21]

How shall we assess this argument? The first premise makes a factual claim, while the second premise states a moral principle. The general intuition underlying this argument is simple enough. If medical workers go on strike, innocent people will be harmed. Since hospitals are nonprofit organizations, such a strike is not felt keenly by management. Moreover, those who feel the adverse effects of the strike are just those whom medical workers claim to be helping, their patients. The withholding of services by medical workers, then, seems to be a case of misfiring: the intended victim, hospital management, is missed and the alleged beneficiary, the patient, is harmed.[22] The factual claim in the first premise seems to be correct. If strikes by medical workers did not produce risks, the general populace would show little concern about them. Strikes cannot be effective unless they cause problems for someone, and it seems clear that it will be patients who will be harmed by medical workers' strikes. But is premise two correct? Initially it seems to be a moral premise that enjoys widespread acceptance; however, its absolute status (as signified by the word "never") can be called into question. It can be argued that there are extreme circumstances in which it is permissible for medical workers to perform actions that will harm patients. In particular, there may be situations in which no matter what the medical worker does, it will harm some patient or other. The residents and interns of Cook County Hospital might have argued, quite plausibly, along these lines. They may have contended that if they withheld their services some of their present patients would suffer, but if they allowed the status quo to persist many of their future patients would be harmed. In a situation like this, no matter what is done patients will be harmed. The second premise is false, then, because it does not allow for situations in which the medical worker must do something that will harm a patient because each alternative open to him or her will have this effect.

It seems, then, that the major arguments given to show that medical workers should neither unionize nor strike are inadequate because they contain doubtful premises.

## ARGUMENTS SUPPORTING UNIONIZATION
## FOR MEDICAL WORKERS

Regarding the implementation of some sort of national health program as inevitable, some medical workers have rallied to the defense of unionization. If a national health program is instituted, it will definitely weaken the financial position of medical workers. Members of the medical establishment believe that their financial status has already been lowered because of such factors as the greater number of third-party forces, the increase of malpractice suits, and the increased dependence of physicians on institutions such as hospitals. To insure that this status is not further eroded, especially if national health insurance becomes a reality, they believe that medical unions must be formed.

One of the leading proponents of unionization for physicians, Dr. Sanford Marcus,[23] presents several different arguments to support his position. Many of his arguments tie the unionization of medical workers to improved patient care. He claims, for example, that there are already many forces interposing themselves between physicians and their patients: insurance companies, the government, and the hospital industry among others. Though their interference may be motivated by a desire to reduce medical costs, in fact their activities threaten to lower the quality of medical care. Physicians' unions, it is argued, can protect the interests of patients by minimizing the interference of these outside forces. Marcus also contends that unions are needed in order to influence legislation affecting the medical profession. Only the collective voice of the profession can be heard; individuals are impotent.

Another of Marcus' arguments appeals directly to financial considerations. Let us call this the merit argument.[24] According to this argument medical workers ought to unionize because without the right to bargain collectively they cannot be sure of earning what they are worth. Marcus even tells us what he believes that physicians are worth. He cites (in 1975) a figure of $100,000 a year. He frequently reminds the reader that this is how much the senior pilots of Delta Air Lines are making. The inference one is invited to draw, of course, is that physicians are worth at least as much as pilots. Marcus' merit argument can be stated as follows.

1. If physicians are salaried employees they may not get what they are worth compared with other professions (such as pilots).
2. What a person is worth is what that person can command on the free market.
3. The market is free only if there are unions and the right to bargain collectively is protected.
4. So in order to get what they are worth, physicians must have a union and the right to bargain collectively.[25]

Marcus does not state premises two and three explicitly. But they seem to be presupposed by what he does say. He assumes, for example, that the $100,000 salary of the Delta Air Lines' pilots is just. But why this is so, he does not say. The only apparent answer is that this is the salary they were able to achieve through the process of collective bargaining. There are, it seems, two major problems with this argument. The first, related to the point just made, is that the free market concept of "worth"—that a person is worth whatever he or she can command on the free market—is not defended. Considerable argument is needed to establish this controversial claim. And it might be noted that one implication of this concept of worth is that Muhammad Ali and Johnny Carson are worth more than any physician. One wonders if Marcus would really accept this. Second, this argument seems to gain whatever appeal it has by equivocating on the term "worth." (To equivocate is to use the same term to mean two different things.) It seems that in the first premise the term "worth" refers to the notion of social worth. That premise seems acceptable only because most people think that physicians contribute at least as much to society as pilots. In the second premise, however, the free market sense of "worth" is employed. But in order to derive the conclusion from the three premises, the term "worth" must be used univocally. Thus Marcus' merit argument seems weak.

Another argument that Marcus advances might be called the incentive argument for the unionization of medical workers.[26] Here Marcus tries to make a direct link between unions for physicians and improved patient care. He suggests that just as it would not be prudent to fly with a disgruntled airplane pilot, so too it would not be advisable to be treated by an unhappy physician. And a physician's happiness is tied directly to his or her pay. The argument may be stated as follows.

1. Patients will receive adequate care only if medical workers are satisfied with their jobs. (A dissatisfied worker is a bad worker).
2. Medical workers will be satisfied with their jobs only if they are receiving a good salary. (If a medical worker's salary is inadequate, he or she will do a bad job.)
3. Medical workers can be insured a good salary only if they have unions and the right to bargain collectively.
4. Therefore, patients will receive adequate care only if medical workers have unions and the right to bargain collectively.

What this argument tells us is that the effort medical workers put forward and the enthusiasm they have for their jobs will be proportionate to how satisfied they are. Moreover, their degree of satisfaction will depend on how well paid they are. And since the public can only insure that medical workers will be well paid by giving them the right to bargain collectively, that is what must be done.

It is important to understand the theoretical foundations of this argument. The moral principle presupposed by the argument is patient consequentialism. The medical worker's only concern should be the well-being of the patient. The argument appeals to certain factual claims which purportedly show that allowing medical workers to unionize is one course of action necessary to insure that patients receive adequate care. It is worth emphasizing that this is a consequentialist argument, not a utilitarian one. It does not counsel us to maximize the good for everyone; rather we are directed to do that which is in the patient's best interests. The consequentialist principle on which the argument is based could, of course, be challenged. That will not be the strategy followed here, however. Instead let us try to cast doubt on the reasons given in the incentive argument to show that the unionization of medical workers is necessary for patients to receive adequate health care.

If adequate health care were otherwise unattainable, then surely medical workers would be given the right to unionize. But why, according to Marcus, are adequate health care and the unionization of medical workers so closely linked? He makes the connection on the basis of several assumptions that are implicit in the first two premises. What is contained in these premises is a certain psychological portrait of the medical worker when he or she is dispensing services. What Marcus suggests is that monetary concerns motivate the medical worker even when he or she is serving the patient. He assumes that a medical worker who is making less than he or she thinks is appropriate will become disgruntled and the treatment of the patients will become sloppy or perfunctory. The medical worker will have the following attitude: Why should I work carefully and diligently when I am not being paid sufficiently or treated fairly.

Once this portrait is stated explicitly, it is evident that it is unrealistic and implausible. And one need not be so naive as to think that medical workers are motivated solely by altruistic considerations in order to cast doubt on this account. It is, of course, true that medical workers are concerned about monetary matters. But to claim that financial considerations weigh heavily on their minds at the time they are serving their patients seems very doubtful. It is more plausible to say that medical workers—and, for that matter, most professionals—have two disparate sides or aspects to their personalities. For lack of a better description, these aspects might be called the "serving" and the "business" sides. Surely a physician performing surgery is not likely to be careless simply because she is dissatisfied with her salary. As Marcus himself notes, most doctors are dedicated people, and they often perform important services gratis.[27] Similarly, it is hard to believe that a nurse will not care about her patients simply because she is being underpaid. There is evidence gathered from some recent interviews which indicates that even among the semiskilled and unskilled medical workers there is a strong degree of commitment to service. In spite of the fact that these people describe their working conditions as bad and their pay as too low, they show a devotion that is rarely matched by workers in other areas.[28] This suggests that when medical workers are serving their patients, their principal concern is the health of those patients and not the financial rewards they will reap. This is not to say, however, that medical workers are unconcerned about monetary matters. When a medical worker is deciding whether to take a new job offer, salary will certainly be a chief consideration. And, if a medical worker were negotiating a new contract, clearly money would be of paramount importance. It seems, then, that there are two distinct sides to the medical professional, and for the most part they are unrelated. Thus Marcus' version of the incentive argument fails because an important claim implicit in the first two premises is false: money does not play the role that he says it does *at the time a medical worker is dispensing services*.

Nonetheless there does seem to be some connection between motivation and pay, and that is why there seems to be something correct about the incentive argument, or at least a modified version of that argument. The connection is simple enough. If physicians, nurses, and other medical workers are not paid well, good people will not be attracted to these fields and as a result patients will suffer. So it is in the interest of all of us to see to it that the various medical professions are sufficiently lucrative to attract the best possible people. In fact, it is often said that it is precisely our failure on this point which has led to there being an excessive number of surgeons and a shortage of primary care physicians or general practitioners. Does granting this show that the incentive argument is correct after all? It does not. As premise three indicates, Marcus assumes that the only way that medical workers can be assured of a satisfactory salary is if they have the power to bargain collectively. Recall that in this context "satisfactory salary" just means a high enough salary to attract good people. So understood, Marcus' assumption is surely false. At the present time there is no shortage of qualified people seeking admission to medical school; the opposite is the case. This must indicate, according to advocates of the incentive argument themselves, that current salaries are quite satisfactory; the incentive is there. Even if a shortage were to develop, and even if this were caused by too low a pay scale, the problem could be rectified without giving medical workers the right to unionize. Society could simply make the financial rewards of the particular profession great enough so that the best people would again be motivated to enter that field. It seems, then, that the general public is sufficiently motivated to see to it that the salary of medical workers is appropriately high. And this shows that premise three of the incentive argument is false. It seems, then, that neither the merit argument nor the incentive argument succeeds.

## UNIONS AND STRIKES:
## SOME FINAL COMMENTS

We shall return to the question of whether medical workers should have the right to bargain collectively. But first, since the topic has been touched upon, let us ask what justification, if any, there is for the fact that physicians receive very high salaries.[29] Among the traditional defenses given to support such high salaries, one states that physicians should be compensated for their long, expensive training. This reason, though, seems very weak. Much of the training that medical students receive is funded by the public (through federal grants, low-interest federal loans, and the like). In addition, residents and interns are paid for their services. Finally, if one includes the years spent in training as working years and averages out the income on this basis, physicians are still compensated much more than most workers. A second defense given for the high salaries received by doctors is that this reflects the burden of high responsibility that they must bear. But this too seems inadequate. There are others who must take on great responsibilities or who must undertake great risks who are not remunerated nearly as well. Police officers and nurses are two good examples. The third, and most common, defense to justify high salaries for doctors suggests that high salaries are needed as incentives. No doubt, salaries must be reasonably high in order to encourage good people to become doctors. But whether they need to be nearly as high as they are is quite another matter. If physicians' salaries were three-quarters what they are now, would far fewer persons seek entry into the medical profession? It seems unlikely that this would happen since the salary would still be much higher than what most people make. Moreover, there are some professions, the position of a university professor, for example, where salaries are relatively low and yet the competition for those positions is very great. A fourth reason given to justify high salaries for physicians is that this reflects the importance of their contribution to the social good compared with other workers. This is probably the most promising defense. It is interesting to note, however, that our society does not employ such a criterion consistently. If it did, surely nurses and police officers would receive more pay and professional athletes, entertainers, and divorce lawyers would receive less. Whether very high salaries for physicians are justified remains an open question. It seems, though, that the traditional defenses are very weak.

Let us return to the question of whether medical workers should be permitted to unionize if national health insurance or socialized medicine becomes a reality. It is plausible to answer this query affirmatively. To support unionization, one does not need arguments of the sort presented by Dr. Marcus. The matter is much simpler. If medical workers are transformed from private entrepreneurs to government employees, they need some means of protecting themselves against the power of their employers. Without a union or the power to bargain collectively, medical workers will have no effective way to make known their grievances. Unacceptable employment conditions may be forced on medical workers if they are not organized. It can be maintained, therefore, that if the government does take over the health care system, in part or completely, then medical workers do have a right to unionize and to bargain collectively. And this right may exist even if the government is not involved in the health care system. The key is whether others have authority and control over medical workers, whether working conditions are established by others. Medical workers have a right to some say in the matter when an employer decides to alter their working conditions. Unions may be a necessary instrument for exercising this right. Certainly given the situation of nurses in hospitals, they have a right to unionize and to bargain collectively. Residents and interns also have this right, it can be argued. Whether they want or need to exercise the right, of course, is another matter.

If medical workers have a right to unionize and to bargain collectively, it is natural to assume that they have the right to strike too, at least in extreme circumstances. After all, what good is the right to bargain collectively if medical workers may not withhold their services? Such an inference, however, may be too quick. If the demands of medical workers could receive a fair hearing, then unions without the right to strike would not be impotent. Some sort of system of binding arbitration might make this possible. A neutral board of arbitors would request that each side submit its proposal for settling the dispute (whether it be about working conditions, pay, or whatever). Each side would agree to abide by the board's ruling. The board would then rule in favor of one side or the other; once the matter is put before the board, no compromising will be done. This encourages each side to present reasonable demands; to do otherwise is to ensure that one will lose. The advantage of this system is that the grievances of medical workers are given a fair hearing and patients are not harmed because of a strike. The greatest difficulty with the system concerns the makeup of the arbitration board. Would it be possible to get a group of people who are neutral and acceptable to each side? If medical workers are included on the board, management may feel cheated. If medical workers are excluded from membership on the board, the union will protest. The problem of the makeup of the arbitration board must still be solved. If it can, though, this seems far preferable to allowing medical workers the right to withhold their services.

If a system of binding arbitration is not feasible, then the right to bargain collectively without the accompanying right to strike would be useless. When, then, would medical workers be justified in withholding their services? One philosopher, Norman Daniels, has argued that the following three conditions must be satisfied if a strike by medical workers is justified.[30] First, a significant part of the medical workers' goals and demands must be directly related to improved patient care. Second, it must be the case that there is no other way to achieve the goals that involves less risk to the general population. All other means of settling the dispute have been tried and failed. Finally, the strike must be aimed at some third-party which has the power to grant to the medical workers the goals they are seeking. When the physicians in California and New York partook in a slowdown in order to protest the costs of malpractice insurance, their activities were aimed at their state legislatures who had the power to regulate such matters. This proposal does not allow for a strike solely for monetary reasons. However, one can imagine extreme circumstances in which such strikes would be justifiable. If medical workers were government employees and grossly underpaid, a strike for pecuniary reasons would be appropriate. With this added qualification, the account just presented seems defensible. A system of binding arbitration is surely preferable. But if it is not workable, the proposal just presented may be the most plausible alternative.

## SUMMARY

In a relatively wealthy society each citizen should have access to adequate health care, or so the view characterized as the liberal position maintains. The conservative, by contrast, argues that medical care should be treated like any other good on the open market: a person is free to purchase whatever health care that he or she regards as worthwhile and affordable. If access to adequate health care is something that a society guarantees to each of its citizens, then it will be necessary to redistribute some of the wealth. Conservatives contend that this forces a person to benefit others and that such a practice is unjustifiable. In order to implement the liberal position, either the government will have to act as a third party and pay medical workers when they serve low income patients or it will have to take over the entire health care system. The conservative claims that because of the possibilities of abuse, the loss of rights, and the increase in cost, neither of these alternatives is acceptable. One who defends the view that equal access to health care is a right must deal with these objections.

Conditions may arise in which medical workers are motivated to unionize. If the government were to take over the entire health care structure, then all medical workers would have reasons to unionize. As things stand now, nurses and medical technicians have grounds for unionizing; whether physicians do is another matter. If medical workers have unions, then the threat that they will withhold their services will be imminent. Some have argued that medical workers should never unionize or strike. To do so, it is claimed, is contrary to the medical worker's professionalism and imposes unjustified risks on patients. Each of these arguments, however, is susceptible to serious objections. Dr. Sanford Marcus has been a vigorous defender of unions for medical workers. It is his contention that medical workers cannot be sure of receiving the salary they deserve and will not be motivated to provide the best service possible unless they are unionized. There are serious difficulties with his arguments too, however. It does seem, though, that if medical workers become government employees (because of the implementation of national health insurance), then they must have some way to protect themselves against their employers and to make known their grievances. The most obvious way to achieve this is through unionization. From this, it need not follow that medical workers have the right to strike. If a fair system of binding arbitration is possible, medical workers can be protected and patients need not be exposed to the risk of strikes. If such a system is not possible, however, then the issue of when it is appropriate for medical workers to strike will be a pressing one.

## CASE STUDY

On February 1, 1980, the registered nurses at Columbia-Presbyterian Medical Center in New York went on strike. The strike ended on February 5, 1980, when, by a vote of 606 to 211, the nurses agreed to accept a new contract. Among the demands made by the nurses were these: nursing and nonnursing functions would be specified and the latter function would be reduced; mandatory overtime work schedules would be reduced; salaries would be increased; and nursing practice committees would be formed. During the strike, intensive care units were staffed and patients who could not be transferred or cared for by nonstriking personnel were attended to. Although the nurses did not get everything they wanted, significant advances were made. It was agreed that there would be a decrease in nonnursing functions and that some would be eliminated. The number of mandatory double shifts required per year was reduced from 49 to 13. They received a 26 percent increase in salary over a three-year period. Their salary at the time was $14,700.[31]

## Discussion Questions

1. Many of the nurses at Columbia–Presbyterian Medical Center indicated that the decision to go on strike was a difficult one, but that personal and professional responsibilities required it. How do you think they would respond to the argument that unionizing conflicts with a medical worker's professional obligations?
2. How do you think these striking nurses might respond to the argument that medical workers should never withhold their services because of the risks that this creates for patients?
3. Of the considerations supporting unions for medical workers discussed in this chapter (Marcus' two arguments and the points raised at the end of this chapter), which do you think these nurses would be most likely to cite in support of their action?
4. Given the information presented, do you think the nurses were justified in going on strike? Explain why or why not.

## SUGGESTIONS FOR FURTHER READING

Norman Daniels, "On the Picket Line: Are Doctors' Strikes Ethical?" *The Hastings Center Report*, Vol. 8 (1978), pp. 24–29.

Barbara Ehrenreich and John Ehrenreich, "The American Health Empire: The System Behind the Chaos," in Thomas A. Mappes and Jane S. Zembaty (eds.), *Biomedical Ethics* (New York: McGraw-Hill Book Company, 1981), pp. 537–544.

Kathleen M. Fenner, *Ethics and Law in Nursing* (New York: D. Van Nostrand Company, 1980), pp. 138–144.

George H. Kieffer, *Bioethics: A Textbook of Issues* (Reading Mass.: Addison-Wesley Publishing Company, 1979), pp. 313–341.

William E. Mann, "Rights, Consequences, and Health Care," in Ronald Munson (ed.), *Intervention and Reflection* (Belmont, Calif.: Wadsworth Publishing Company, 1979), pp. 473–480.

Robert Nozick, *Anarchy, State, and Utopia* (New York: Basic Books, 1974).

Gene Outka, "Social Justice and Equal Access to Health Care," *The Journal of Religious Ethics*, Vol. 2 (1974), pp. 11–32.

John Rawls, *A Theory of Justice* (Cambridge, Mass.: Harvard University Press, 1971).

Robert M. Sade, "Medical Care as a Right," in *Intervention and Reflection*, pp. 457–462.

James P. Sterba (ed.), *Justice: Alternative Political Perspectives* (Belmont, Calif: Wadsworth Publishing Company, 1980).

## NOTES

1. For this way of explaining rights, see Joel Feinberg, *Social Philosophy* (Englewood Cliffs, New Jersey: Prentice-Hall, 1973), pp. 56–58. Many of the distinctions that I draw here are explained carefully by Feinberg. See especially, Chapter Four.
2. Though I am not presenting their views there, in philosophical circles the best known defenses of the liberal and conservative theories of distributive justice are, respectively, John Rawls, *A Theory of Justice* (Cambridge, Mass.: Harvard University Press, 1971) and Robert Nozick, *Anarchy, State, and Utopia* (New York: Basic Books, 1974). See also, James P. Sterba (ed.), *Justice: Alternative Political Perspectives* (Belmont, Calif.: Wadsworth Publishing Company, 1980).
3. The idea that I present here is taken from Rawls, *A Theory of Justice.* However, the reader should realize that my presentation is a gross oversimplification. Rawls' views are far more complicated and defended by many cogent arguments.
4. Again, this is an embarrassingly crude presentation of the conservative theory. I have presented only those elements necessary in order to understand the dispute concerning the right to health care. For a full-blown defense of the conservative view, see Nozick, *Anarchy, State, and Utopia*, Chapter Seven.
5. For most of the points made here, I am indebted to George H. Kieffer, *Bioethics: A Textbook of Issues* (Reading, Mass.: Addison-Wesley Publishing Company, 1979), pp. 313–341.
6. On this point, see Kieffer, *Bioethics: A Textbook of Issues*, p. 314.
7. At least one philosopher, though, seems to construe the right to health care as a negative right. Richard Warner, in *Morality in Medicine* (Sherman Oaks, Calif.: Alfred Publishing Company, 1980), p. 121, says that the right to health care is simply a right that others should not interfere with one's health care.
8. The argument for the liberal view that will be examined here is presented by Gene Outka, "Social Justice and Equal Access to Health Care," *The Journal of Religious Ethics*, Vol. 2 (1974), pp. 11–32.
9. Outka states this criterion is a more complex way: "To each according to his contribution in satisfying whatever is freely desired by others in the open marketplace of supply and demand." See "Social Justice and Equal Access to Health Care," p. 19.
10. See Outka, "Social Justice and Equal Access to Health Care," pp. 23–25.
11. Sketches of these programs are offered by George H. Kieffer in *Bioethics: A Textbook of Issues*, pp. 324–328. My account here borrows heavily from Kieffer, though there are some differences.
12. This second criticism is discussed by Thomas S. Szasz, "The Right to Health," in Samuel Gorovitz *et al.* (eds.), *Moral Problems in Medicine* (Englewood Cliffs, New Jersey: Prentice-Hall, 1976), pp. 475–478.
13. For a general statement of the effect the state's taking over the medical apparatus will have on the physician-patient relationship, see Szasz, "The Right to Health," p. 478.
14. A case of this sort is presented and discussed by Robert M. Veatch, *Case Studies in Medical Ethics* (Cambridge, Mass.: Harvard University Press, 1977), pp. 107–110.

15. This same point is made, though in a different context, by Kathleen M. Fenner, *Ethics and Law in Nursing* (New York: D. Van Nostrand Company, 1980), p. 139.
16. Much of the information in this section is taken from the excellent article by Norman Daniels, "On the Picket Line: Are Doctors' Strikes Ethical?" *The Hastings Center Report*, Vol. 8 (1978), pp. 24–29.
17. The reasons for the strike by the interns and residents are discussed by Daniels, "On the Picket Line," p. 24. The case of the strike by nurses is dealt with by Fenner, *Ethics and Law in Nursing*, p. 141.
18. See Fenner, *Ethics and Law in Nursing*, p. 140.
19. The discussion here is based on Daniels, "On the Picket Line," pp. 24–25.
20. This argument is presented (in a slightly different form) and discussed by Daniels, "On the Picket Line," pp. 25–26.
21. This argument concludes that medical workers should not strike. It says nothing against forming unions. It is assumed, though, that unions without the right to strike are virtually powerless (with one possible exception to be noted later) and so the two can be linked together.
22. On this point, see Fenner, *Ethics and Law in Nursing*, p. 141.
23. See Sanford A. Marcus, "The Purpose of Unionization in the Medical Profession," *International Journal of Health Services*, Vol. 5 (1975), pp. 37–42 and Marcus, "The Time Has Come to Bargain for Higher Incomes," *Medical Economics*, Vol. 52 (1975), pp. 204–214.
24. The argument is sketched informally by Marcus in "The Time Has Come to Bargain for Higher Incomes," p. 207. For the label I give to this argument as well as some of the critical points I make, I am indebted to Daniels, "On the Picket Line," pp. 26–27.
25. Two points should be noted here. First, Marcus restricts his discussion to unions for physicians. There is no reason, however, why the arguments cannot be extended to cover all medical workers. Second, Marcus does not advocate that physicians strike to achieve their ends. Rather he favors activities designed to disrupt the bureaucracy that is trying to interfere with the medical profession, activities such as refusing to fill out forms involved in third-party payments.
26. Marcus states this argument in "The Time Has Come to Bargain for Higher Incomes," p. 214. The label I give to this argument is suggested by Daniels, "On the Picket Line," p. 27. The discussion of this argument is taken from my paper, "The Incentive Argument for the Unionization of Medical Workers," *Journal of Medical Ethics*, Vol. 5 (1979), pp. 182–184.
27. Marcus, "The Time Has Come to Bargain for Higher Incomes," p. 209.
28. Barbara Ehrenreich and John Ehrenreich, "Hospital Workers: Class Conflicts in the Making," *International Journal of Health Services*, Vol. 5 (1975), pp. 44–45.
29. In my brief discussion here I follow the account of Daniels, "On the Picket Line," p. 28.
30. Daniels, "On the Picket Line," p. 29.
31. See the *American Journal of Nursing*, March 1980, pp. 377 and 388, and Ruth Korn, "Nurses United: One Staff's Decision to Strike," *American Journal of Nursing*, December 1980, pp. 2218–2221.

# 8

# Obtaining and Allocating Scarce Medical Resources

This chapter will focus on two moral problems that arise when the demand for certain medical resources far exceeds the supply. First, what is the best way to obtain more of this resource? And second, how should this resource be distributed when, because of scarcity, each person's needs cannot be fulfilled?

Medical resources can be divided into two types, *human* resources and *nonhuman* resources. Each of these categories designates the origin of the resource. Human resources are obtained directly from human beings. Examples of human medical resources include blood and organs for transplantation, such as kidneys and hearts. Nonhuman medical resources are either made by human beings or are found in nature. Examples of nonhuman medical resources include drugs, artificial organs, dialysis machines, respirators, and the like. When discussing the issue of *allocating* scarce medical resources, this distinction does not seem to be very important. It seems that the same principles should apply whether the scarce resource to be distributed is human or nonhuman. When talking about how to *obtain* scarce resources, however, the distinction does seem important. In principle, the question of obtaining nonhuman medical resources seems to be a simple one. Making a nonhuman medical resource more plentiful would seem to be a matter of spending more time and money and developing more ingenuity. There may, of course, be serious moral questions raised here, especially if the money to be invested is public money. But here the focus will be on moral questions raised in obtaining human medical resources.

Human medical resources can be further distinguished, depending on how the donor of the resource is affected. In some cases, for example, when giving blood, the donor is living and his or her loss is temporary. In other cases the donor is living but his or her loss is permanent. A person who donates a kidney falls into this second category. Finally, some human resources can be obtained only when the donor is dead. To cite an obvious example, hearts can be obtained only when the donor has died. There is some overlap in these categories, of course. Kidneys can be obtained from living donors or from cadavers. In our discussion of obtaining human medical resources, the focus will be on two of these categories: the case in which the donor is dead and the case in which the donor is alive and his or her loss is temporary. This is not to say that the other category is unimportant; it is quite important. The typical case that falls under this category is when a person decides to donate one of his or her kidneys to a relative. Moral questions about this sort of case focus on what is required of the would-be donor. Can someone be required to make a sacrifice of this sort? And isn't there a great danger that the would-be donor will be coerced into giving his or her kidney to the relative in need? Although they are important, these questions will be ignored for now.

## OBTAINING CADAVER ORGANS

Since the advent of transplantation, cadaver organs are valuable medical resources. Now hearts, kidneys, and other organs from the newly dead might be used to save lives. At the present time to obtain cadaver organs for transplantation, society relies principally on donations. And it can be said without exaggeration that this system is not working very well. Consider, for example, the need for kidneys. It has been estimated that thousands of those who die from kidney failure each year could be helped with a transplant.[1] It is true, of course, that the chances of benefiting from a kidney transplant are greater if the donor is a living relative. But kidneys from cadavers still have proven to be quite valuable. Similar things can be said about the unavailability of hearts. Though the survival rate of those who receive a heart transplant is considerably less than those who have a transplanted kidney, nevertheless such organs are useful. Again it is estimated that thousands could be helped were hearts from the newly dead available.[2] Since one of the major objectives of medical practice is to save lives and since many more lives can be saved if more organs are available for transplantation, it seems that there is an obligation to find a way to secure a greater number of suitable cadaver organs.

What sort of policy should our society adopt for obtaining cadaver organs? There are at least three possibilities that should be examined.[3] To acquire organs from the dead, society might adopt a *giving* policy, a *trading* policy, or a *taking* policy. Let us examine each of these. A giving policy, just as the name suggests, relies totally on donations. While a person is living, he or she gives permission to the appropriate authorities to take any of his or her organs which can be used upon death. The giving policy has been adopted in the United States. In order to provide some unity and clarity to state laws, the Uniform Anatomical Gift Act was drafted in 1968. Now all fifty states have adopted the major provisions of this act. One of the major purposes of this act is to allow the wishes of the deceased to donate his or her organs to stand even if the next-of-kin protests. The act's five major provisions follow below.[4]

1. Any person over 18-years-old may donate all or part of his or her body for research or transplantation purposes.
2. If a person has not made a donation before his or her death, that person's next-of-kin may do so unless it is known that the deceased had an objection.
3. If the person has made such a gift it cannot be revoked by his or her relatives.
4. If there is more than one person of the same degree of kinship, the gift from relatives shall not be accepted if any of them has an objection.
5. The gift can be authorized if the person carries a card or if written or verbal communication has been recorded by a relative.

This is an outline of the giving policy currently in operation in the United States today. It enables a person or his or her relatives to donate organs upon death.

The giving policy, no matter how it is set up, has certain advantages. Most importantly, this policy respects an individual's right to autonomy and freedom. It recognizes that a person's body is his or her property and may be used as desired. If a person wants to be generous and donate his or her body to medicine, that is an option that may be exercised. There are certain difficulties with the giving policy, however. First and foremost, it is not working. Too few people are offering their bodies to medicine. If most people had religious or moral objections to having parts of their bodies used after they die, then this would not be a serious objection. It would simply be an indication that many people disapprove of the use of cadaver organs for transplantation. However, the evidence suggests that most people favor such a practice. Not only that, but a 1968 Gallup Poll showed that 70 percent of the adults in the United States approved of giving their own organs after death.[5] In spite of this and the enactment of the Uniform Anatomical Gift Act, very few people have donated their own organs or those of relatives. Perhaps people are just not motivated. Whatever the reason, the giving policy is not working. In order to make the giving policy work, it would have to be much more aggressive, and this is the second objection. Pressure would have to be exerted on people. Among other problems such an aggressive program would create is that it would put too great of a burden on those who are very ill. Pressure would be exerted on persons at a time when they are least able to resist or to deal with it. Finally, a giving policy such as that embodied in the Uniform Anatomical Gift Act has the disadvantage of requiring family approval at the time of death, the time when the family is least likely to give that approval. This is especially problematic when one realizes that the most suitable organ donors are teenagers who have died in an accident. Their organs are much more useful than those of a person who has suffered from a debilitating disease. But their parents are likely to be in shock and perhaps they feel guilty too. In any case, they are not likely to approve. The giving policy, then, has not attracted enough donors and does not enable us to secure the organs of the most suitable donors.

The trading policy is the second approach that a society might try. Such a policy is set up to induce people to allow their organs to be used when they die. As an incentive, these potential "donors" are offered something in return.[6] What they are offered depends on the program. One obvious incentive would be some sort of financial compensation. If a person signs a document agreeing to contribute his or her organs upon death, then that person will be paid a given amount of money. A society could provide a different incentive, though. It could pool all cadaver organs for transplantation and allow only those who have themselves agreed to contribute their organs to have access to the organs as a medical resource. In this latter setup a person would be trading usable organs upon death in exchange for the right to use any available organs that might be needed while alive. Either version of the trading policy, however, is open to objections.

The first form of the trading policy would probably be too costly. In order to induce people to contribute their organs, the cash payment will have to be reasonably large. And since the pool of potential donors must be large (because not everyone's organs will be usable), the total cost will be significant. In addition, this version of the trading policy will put most of the burden of contributing organs on the poor. They, after all, will be the persons most motivated to trade for pay. Finally, it seems likely that a trade-for-pay system could be easily abused. For example, a person who had already received his or her reward might then claim to have converted to a religion which requires that one be buried intact. This will put policy makers in a difficult position. Either they will have to act against a person's alleged religious beliefs (and undoubtedly be bombarded with law suits from relatives and those of the same religious sect) or they will have to set up the system so that the trade is not irrevocable (thus allowing for the possibility of abuses).

The other version of the trading policy is not open to these objections, but it too seems far from desirable. There is something appealing about making organs for transplantation available only to those who have agreed to make their own organs available. It appeals to one's sense of fairness. A person should not expect to reap benefits unless or she is willing to bear a fair share of the burdens. There are, however, both practical and moral problems with such a system. On the practical side, when must a person declare his or her intentions to contribute? Obviously children and teenagers must be allowed access to the organs even though they have not agreed to give. And suppose a person does not agree to contribute until that person realizes it is very likely that he or she will need an organ soon. If this is allowed, it may turn out that the vast majority of the donors are persons who are old and ill. Thus the supply of available organs will be inadequate. On the moral side, as a policy for distributing health care, this strikes many as much too crass. In particular, suppose that at a given time there is only one person who needs an available organ for transplantation. Without this organ, the person will die. No one else needs the organ and if it is not used soon it will go to waste. It seems foolish and immoral to refuse to allow this person the use of the organ, even if this person has not agreed to contribute an organ. Neither version of the trading policy, then, seems plausible.

The third policy for obtaining cadaver organs for transplantation is the taking policy. A society that adopts this policy salvages any of a person's useful organs upon his or her death unless that person has explicitly requested that this not be done. The taking policy has a number of advantages. First, such a system will greatly increase the available supply of organs. In fact, the taking system will provide as many suitable organs as can be obtained. Second, such a system will be efficient and not very costly. Since the organs will be obtained free, the only cost of the system will be setting it up so that organs can be taken immediately upon a person's death. And, it might be claimed, this system respects a person's autonomy in that it allows him or her to be buried intact by so stating that desire. There are, however, some serious objections to a taking policy. First, some have contended that this puts an unfair burden on a patient in the hospital who is suffering. Such a person must state any objections that he or she has at this most unfortunate time. Second, the policy of routinely taking organs will deprive people of the opportunity to exercise the virtue of generosity.[7] If someone voluntarily gives something to another person, the action has a moral quality that it lacks if the person is forced to contribute. If the taking system is instituted, no one will have the opportunity to donate generously his or her organs. The state would seize those organs unless the person had previously protested. In such a society one of the noblest acts that one can perform is not open to people. The third objection looks at the long-range consequences that might ensue if such a policy is adopted. It is very dangerous to allow the state to assume that the parts of its citizens' bodies belong to it (unless the citizens declare otherwise).[8] If the state is permitted to interfere in such an essential matter, what limit can there be on its power? Surely if a society values freedom, it must allow an individual to control his or her own body, including what happens to it after the person's death.

There are, then, serious objections to each of the three policies. The trading policy seems to be the least acceptable of the three. And the objections raised against the taking policy appear to be quite strong. Recently, however, the taking policy has been defended against these objections.[9] Consider the objection that the taking policy will put too much pressure on those who are seriously ill because it forces them to register their protests at a time when they are vulnerable. The taking policy need not cause such a burden. If the policy is adopted, it will be a public policy of which people are (or should be) aware. So if a person has religious objections to having organs removed after death, as apparently Jehovah's Witnesses and Orthodox Jews do, that person will be able to state those objections well in advance. It seems likely, in fact, that a free society which institutes such a program will not only permit persons to be buried intact if they wish, but will make a form readily available to them to declare their objections.

Turning to the second objection, it is true that the taking policy denies people the opportunity to exercise the virtue of generosity (with respect to the giving of their organs). However, the fact of the matter is that under the giving policy very few people are being generous. It would be better to live in a world in which all of the cadaver organs needed were available because people donated them. But that is not the world in which we live. When people in fact are not giving their organs, then this objection to the taking policy seems feeble.

The third objection warns us to consider carefully how much power the taking policy gives to the state. This is an important warning that should not be ignored. It does not follow, however, that it would be irrational to give this power to the state. It may be in each person's self-interest to support the taking policy. It might be regarded as a trade off of sorts. A person gives up the right to say what happens to his or her body after death. In return, that person will have a much better chance of receiving lifesaving organs if they are needed. This seems like a reasonable trade to make. Nevertheless great care must be taken to insure that the state does not abuse this power; and the development of the needed safeguards may be difficult.

It may be desirable to have limits on the taking policy. In particular, it has been argued that the routine salvaging of organs should be limited to lifesaving organs, that is, organs which, when transplanted, offer good prospects for relief from death now.[10] Consider an example. The success in transplanting kidneys is very good, and so kidneys should be taken if they are needed. Perhaps hearts will qualify too. Lungs and livers will not qualify, though. Someday, though, with the advancement of medical science, they probably will qualify. Of course, to make these advances experiments must be done, and this requires that some of these organs be available. To obtain such organs, it would be better to rely on donations. Here is an area in which people will have the opportunity to exercise the virtue of generosity. Adopting this version of the taking policy does emphasize that there are definite limits on how the state may legitimately use its power.

At least one other objection to any version of the taking policy must be considered. One of the real worries about such a policy concerns the possibility of abuse on the part of medical workers. A physician may be tempted to hasten the death of a patient whose prognosis is poor if he or she has an organ which might save the life of another patient.[11] Or a seriously ill patient who is being treated in the emergency room may be regarded, consciously or unconsciously, as a resource for saving the life of another patient. This is a worrisome consideration that should not be taken too lightly. There may be no way to eliminate completely this danger. Perhaps it can be minimized, though, if we require that a person whose organs are going to be used be declared dead by at least two other physicians not connected with the patient who needs the organs. This at least eliminates the problem that a physician's judgment may be clouded because of a desire to save his or her own patient.

Can anything be said to defuse the objections to the giving policy? There is definitely a shortage of organs for transplantation. More lives could be saved if more organs were available. Unless people become far more altruistic than they now are, this shortage is likely to persist. Even advocates of the giving policy acknowledge this. If the giving policy is to be defended, therefore, it will have to be at a more fundamental level. It might be argued, for example, that the taking policy inappropriately forces a person to benefit another. Statutes that require this are usually called good samaritan laws. Those who oppose such laws hold that the proper function of the state is to protect people against aggressors. It is appropriate for the government to prevent a person from harming another. But for the state to compel a person to bestow benefits upon another is inappropriate, the argument goes. And the taking policy would be forcing a person (after death) to benefit another. The giving policy, by contrast, appropriately recognizes that bestowing benefits is an act of charity that must be freely chosen by individuals. Those who share the ideal of a very limited state will probably find this defense of the giving policy persuasive. Others may find the advantages of the taking policy more convincing.

## OBTAINING RENEWABLE MEDICAL RESOURCES

Renewable medical resources are obtained from living human beings and their loss is temporary. The best known example of this sort of resource is blood. Bone marrow is another example of a renewable medical resource. Blood is obviously a valuable medical resource. Because of the following factors, blood can also be a scarce medical resource.[12] First, not everyone can safely give blood. Some cannot serve as donors because it will adversely affect their own health; others cannot because they would transmit a disease to the recipient of their blood. Second, human blood deteriorates. Some parts of human blood can be saved (as a useful medical resource) for only about three weeks. Third, not only must blood be available, but the right type must be available. A mismatch of types can be lethal. And since some blood types are very rare, there is a natural shortage.

What sort of social policy or policies should be adopted for obtaining a renewable medical resource such as blood? There are at least four possibilities that deserve some consideration. Each of these policies will be listed and then described in more detail. One policy that might be adopted for obtaining blood is the *free market system*. In the free market system people are paid for contributing blood. In such a system, of course, free donations will be accepted; but persons will be paid for contributing blood if they wish. A second policy is the *donorship system*. In this system society's entire supply of blood comes from the voluntary contributions of people. No economic incentives are provided at all. A third policy is called the *taxation system*. In this system each person who is medically able to do so will be required to contribute blood. How often each person is required to contribute will depend on how many able contributors there are and how much blood is needed. No one, of course, will be forced to contribute so frequently that it will create a medical hazard for that person. A fourth policy for obtaining blood is called the *penalty system*. A society that adopts this policy obtains at least part of its blood from persons who have been convicted of some minor offense. For example, instead of fining a person for exceeding the speed limit, a judge may order him or her to contribute a pint of blood. Judge Irving Goldblatt of Holyoke, Massachusetts, actually issued such an order in 1978, though of course this is not a general policy in the United States.

When confronted with these different policies, how should people choose among them? What criteria should be appealed to in assessing these different social policies? In choosing among these different systems, at least the following criteria should be employed: the cost of the system, the quality of blood obtained by the system, the efficiency of the system, and the moral acceptability of the system. Cost is a simple enough criterion. If one system can obtain the same quantity of a scarce resource as a competing system for less money, then if all other things are equal the less costly system is the better one. The quality of blood that a given policy attracts is also very important. Because many diseases can be transmitted through the blood, it is important that a system does not attract the so-called "bad blood." An efficient system involves a minimal amount of waste. This is important when blood is the medical resource because, as was noted earlier, parts of the blood can only be preserved for approximately three weeks. Finally, there might be moral objections to some policies, either because of the inherent nature of the policy or because of consequences of it, and this must be taken into account in choosing among the competing systems.

Let us begin by using these four criteria to compare the free market system and the donorship system. Much has been written on this topic.[13] There was a time when the free market system was used by the United States to obtain much of its blood, while the donorship system was employed in Great Britain. Each system had its defenders and critics. If the criterion of cost is used to compare these two systems, it appears to be no contest. Clearly the free market system is the more costly of the two. There are costs involved with each system, of course. The machinery must be set up for taking in and processing the blood. But there is an obvious additional cost in the free market system: the contributor is paid. Of course, those defending the free market system might argue that unless a financial incentive is provided, the supply of blood will not be great enough. If the donorship system can attract an adequate supply, however, it clearly has an advantage over the free-market system with regard to cost.

Let us turn next to the quality of blood gathered by each policy. Will either the free market policy or the donorship policy have an advantage over the other with regard to this criterion? A brief comment on the problem of "bad blood" is in order here. A major problem is that certain forms of hepatitis can be transmitted from the carrier contributor to the patient who receives his or her blood. And there is no test that can reliably detect the carriers of certain types of hepatitis. Thus the honesty of the contributor with respect to his or her health, medical history, drug habits, and the like is essential. The recipient's life may be endangered if the contributor is not truthful, especially when answering questions about his or her medical history. What sort of arrangements, then, encourage contributors to be truthful? In comparing different policies in this regard, the motives of the contributors must be taken into account.

Consider first the free market system. Persons who sell their blood are apparently in great need of money; note how little they receive for a pint of blood. And if a person is contributing blood because of a desperate need for money, that person will have a strong motive to conceal any medical problems that might disqualify him or her from being a contributor. Thus a person who has had hepatitis but who needs the money will be inclined to lie. By contrast, in the donorship system it would appear that the contributor's motives are altruistic—the person simply wants to help others. If that is the case, then contributors in the donorship system will be motivated to be truthful in answering questions about their health and their medical history. They will not want a recipient to receive their blood if it will have harmful effects. Hence it is argued that the quality of blood obtained by the donorship system will be superior to that obtained by the free market system. This point is reinforced when one considers that most of those who sell their blood will be poor, and the incidence of hepatitis (and other diseases) is higher among the poor than it is in the general population at large. The probability that the free market system will attract more bad blood is higher, then, because contributors in the donorship system will presumably come from all segments of the population.

What about the efficiency of the free market and donorship systems? When the free market system of the United States was compared with the donorship policy as it operated in England and Wales, it was estimated that the American system wasted ten times as much blood as the British system, proportionately. This suggests, then, that the free market system is much less efficient than the donorship system. The crucial question, however, is *why* did the United States' system waste more blood. To show that the free market system is inherently less efficient, a person would have to demonstrate that the *reason* the free market system is more wasteful is because it pays for blood.[14] And it is hard to see how this can be shown. Some have suggested that the reason the United States system was more wasteful was that the price it charged for blood did not adequately reflect its scarcity; thus people were encouraged to use it more frequently than necessary and in a wasteful manner. It is even possible that people in the United States are by nature more wasteful than others, regardless of the system employed. So the figures cited above do not prove that the donorship system is more efficient than the free market system.

Finally, let us turn to the criterion of moral acceptability. Are there moral objections to either the free market system or the donorship system? Defenders of the donorship system have pointed to two considerations to support the claim that the free market system is morally inferior to the donorship system. First, it is contended that the free market system exploits the poor. In such a system, it is argued, most contributors are either poor or from a captive population (for example, prisoners). Some of the frequent contributors are those who are temporarily poor, such as graduate students, medical students, and the like. Others are those whose economic status is more permanent. But in either case the rich are, in effect, buying blood from the poor. Even if this is acknowledged as a fact, there are two different responses that might be made to it.[15] The critics of the free market system—those who object to that system on moral grounds—hold that a person should never take advantage of another because of his or her social position. If a person does anything, it should be to change those bad conditions. Those who object to the free market system because it exploits the poor seem to be committed to this position. On the other hand, those who defend the free market system might maintain that when conditions are poor or substandard, what ought to be done is to make the best of a bad situation. And, the defender argues, this is what the free market system does. Blood is a medical necessity that can be safely obtained from people. If paying people for blood enables us to obtain an adequate supply and improve (slightly) the condition of the poor, then this is all the better. Critics of the free market system lament the fact that in a society that adopts such a policy the burden of supplying blood is borne almost entirely by the poor. Defenders of the system rejoice at the fact that this enables some of the poor to improve their position, though ever so slightly.

The second point that critics make to show that the free market system is morally inferior to the donorship system is that a purely voluntary system encourages altruism, while the free market system or a mixed system (in which at least some are paid for contributing blood) discourages altruism.[16] The contention here is that experiments show that in situations calling for an altruistic response, people are more inclined to respond altruistically if they have recently witnessed someone else behaving altruistically. Applying this to the issue of how best to obtain blood, critics have made the following points. If it is known that some people will be paid for contributing blood, very few will be motivated to give their blood freely. On the other hand, if people see others giving blood, they will be inclined to do so themselves. As a moral objection to the free market system, this point appeals to the alleged consequences of adopting that policy. Presumably the idea is that of two societies, the one with more altruism is better, everything else being equal. And since the donorship system promotes further altruism while the free market system does not, the donorship system is morally preferable. If the factual assumption underlying this objection is correct, this provides an argument not merely for adopting the donorship system, but rather for publicizing the fact that people are giving.

Our discussion of the free market and donorship systems might be concluded by noting that though today the United States still employs a mixed system, most blood is donated. It has been reported that only about five percent of whole blood is paid for in the United States.[17] Still, the controversy about the appropriateness of buying blood continues. In December of 1979 the Food and Drug Administration investigated the Community Blood and Plasma Service of Winston-Salem, North Carolina. Community Blood buys plasma from contributors. The charges leveled against this company are quite similar to those made against the free market system in general. Questions were raised about the contributors, for example. It was contended that many had been previously rejected because of problems such as alcoholism and drug abuse. It was also charged, in effect, that the company exploited the poor. A number of those who sold their plasma were "overbled," that is, they were allowed to contribute too much blood and more frequently than is medically advisable. And in at least one case the wrong red blood cells were returned to a contributor.[18] It was also claimed that those who sold their plasma were not adequately informed of the possible dangers of doing so. All of this has led many to be very suspicious about a system that pays for any of the blood that it obtains.

Employing the same four criteria, let us see how the taxation system fares. This is a policy which requires each medically able person to contribute blood periodically. Certainly one of the chief advantages of this system is that an adequate supply of blood will be available. In fact, this system will supply as much blood as any system can safely obtain. Consider now the cost of such a system. The blood it obtains, of course, is free. There will be, however, costs involved in setting up the system. A bureaucratic structure will be necessary to insure that each medically able person contributes when his or her turn comes. The taxation system will certainly cost more than the donorship system, but how much more is unclear. How efficient will a taxation system be? Will too much blood be wasted? With so many people contributing, the system will have to be set up so that the supply of blood comes in evenly and not all at once (because red cells deteriorate after three weeks). Presumably, though, this can be taken into account when the system is set up. Suppose that each person who is able must contribute once a year. The system might then be arranged so that each must donate on his or her birthday. An arrangement of this sort can minimize waste because of deterioration.

Initially it might be thought that the taxation system would attract more bad blood than any of the other systems because it requires each person to contribute unless he or she is not a suitable donor. The major problem, of course, is that some diseases, such as hepatitis, can be transmitted by blood and one cannot detect this simply by testing the blood. But is it unlikely that would-be contributors would be honest if the taxation policy were enacted? If the taxation were implemented, contributing blood would probably be regarded by most as a burden. Thus people would be motivated to avoid this burden if possible. For this reason, people who have had medical problems in the past would probably be honest when they were asked about their history. It is not likely, then, that the taxation system would attract too much bad blood. Ironically, suitable donors would probably lie to try to avoid the burden of contributing blood.

Finally, what can be said about the moral acceptability of the taxation system? One of the strong points of this policy is that it distributes the burden of supplying blood as equally as possible. Certainly this system does not exploit the poor. There may be moral objections to this system, though. Some will argue that it is inappropriate for the government to force some people to benefit others. As was seen earlier, such persons claim that the state should restrict itself to preventing harm. And, the critic might continue, taking a person's blood is even worse than taking several hours of labor, as is done when people are forced to pay taxes. A second objection that might be raised against this policy is reminiscent of one made against the policy of taking cadaver organs: a system that forces each person to contribute denies a person the opportunity to be altruistic and thus diminishes the moral quality of an individual act. The task of tallying the pluses and minuses of the taxation system and reaching a judgment concerning its ultimate acceptability will be left to the reader.

Let us turn finally to the penalty system. This policy advocates collecting blood instead of a fine from those who are found guilty of misdemeanors (and who are medically suitable contributors). If such a policy were adopted, it would have to serve as a supplement to some other system: it alone presumably could not collect enough blood. In a society which had adopted the taxation system, the penalty policy would be superfluous. After all, the taxation system is set up so that society will have all of the blood it needs. The question of adopting the penalty system, then, arises only in a society whose principal means of obtaining blood is either the donorship system or the free market system. There is no reason to believe that the cost of this system would create any problem. And efficiency will cause no special problems either: the penalty system will be just as efficient as the system it supplements. Would the penalty policy be more likely to attract bad blood? Initially one might think that it would not. There is no reason to think that persons who have had hepatitis are more likely to commit misdemeanors than anyone else. The motivations of those who will be contributors, however, must be examined.

Under the penalty system contributing a pint of blood would be an alternative to a fine. Someone who is medically unable to contribute blood will pay a fine. If someone is guilty of violating the speed limit and cannot give blood, that person will pay a fine. Now suppose that a very poor person is convicted of exceeding the speed limit. And suppose that this person has had hepatitis. Paying the fine may well be beyond this person's means. Hence such a person will be motivated to lie about his or her medical history because giving a pint of blood will be easier than paying a fine. And because the incidence of hepatitis is highest among the poor, the danger of obtaining bad blood if the penalty system is adopted is great. Whether the penalty system is morally acceptable depends on what sort of punishment for crimes is permissible. Is forcing someone to contribute blood an appropriate way of having him repay his debt to society? Taking blood from a person because of his or her wrongdoing may strike many as inappropriate. But what, in principle, is the difference between taking a person's blood or taking ten days of his or her freedom? And if contributing blood is offered as one of several options (the other choices being a fine or imprisonment), are the criminal's rights being violated? These are questions which those opposing the penalty system on moral grounds must answer.

This, then, is a brief look at four different policies that present themselves as candidates when a society is deciding how to obtain renewable medical resources. If an adequate supply of the resource in question can be obtained through the donorship system, then it would seem that appeals to cost, the quality of the product obtained, and moral considerations would overwhelmingly favor that policy. If an adequate supply cannot be obtained through a giving policy, however, then the other systems must be examined more seriously.

## THE ALLOCATION OF SCARCE MEDICAL RESOURCES

As has been noted, some medical resources are valuable and scarce. All sorts of medical resources are potentially scarce. This includes machinery such as dialysis machines and respirators, drugs, human resources such as blood and organs for transplantation, and the time of the medical worker. Often these are lifesaving medical resources. When these resources are scarce, the demand or need for them exceeds the supply. Under these circumstances someone must decide who among the candidates will receive the scarce medical resource. This is the moral problem in these situations. In dealing with this moral problem, several questions must be answered. What criterion or criteria should be used in deciding who receives scarce medical resources? And who should decide who receives these resources? Should the decision be made by the physician, all of the medical workers involved, or by a committee made up in part of laymen? It should be stressed here that the decision to be made is a moral and not a medical decision. It should also be emphasized that moral problems such as these are unavoidable.[19] That this is a moral decision perhaps explains why recently a number of hospitals have formed ethics committees, composed at least in part of laymen, to deal with such issues.

It is tempting to think that the problem of allocating scarce medical resources will disappear when technology becomes sufficiently advanced. To think this, however, is a mistake. Given the nature of advancement in medicine, there will always be some scarce resource or other. Typically, when new discoveries are made the resource in question is expensive and difficult to produce. Improvements may be made with respect to that resource so that it is no longer scarce, but another will come along. Depending on the society and its stage of development, the scarce resource may be penicillin, dialysis machines, blood, organs for transplantation, or simply the time the medical worker has to give to his or her patients. But though the particular good to be allocated may change, the moral problem will always exist.

Speaking generally, there are two competing criteria that have been suggested to serve as the basis for allocating scarce medical resources. One appeals to considerations of social utility or to the social worth of the candidates. According to this criterion, society should allocate its scarce medical resources to those who make the most valuable contributions. Thus, for example, it might be maintained that physicians should be saved ahead of common laborers, that nurses should receive treatment before maids, and that engineers should be selected ahead of barbers. The other criterion for allocating scarce medical resources might be called the lottery method. According to this criterion, each person should have an equal opportunity to receive the scarce medical resource. This end can best be achieved by using the lottery method. Just as the name suggests, each person who needs the resource will have his or her name put in the lottery. The number of names to be drawn will depend on how much of the resource is available. No judgments of social worth will be made. Each person will be considered and the winners will be determined by the luck of the draw. Each of these methods of distributing scarce medical resources will be examined in detail later.

To introduce this topic, let us discuss one case in which a committee was actually formed which formulated criteria for allocating a valuable medical resource. This took place at the Swedish Hospital in Seattle, Washington, in 1962.[20] The scarce medical resource in this case was dialysis machines for victims of kidney failure. The number of persons who needed the treatment was greater than the available supply at the Swedish Hospital. A committee of laymen was selected to choose among the applicants. Members of the committee remained anonymous to protect them from public pressures. An effort was made to have many different elements of the community represented on the committee. In 1963, for example, the committee was composed of two physicians, a banker, a lawyer, a homemaker, a labor leader, and a clergyman. (The idea behind this sort of representation was to prevent skewed or prejudicial judgments that might result if only a few segments of the community were involved.) Given the sorts of decisions that were to be made, this was literally a life-or-death committee. The committee adopted a version of the theory which distributes scarce medical resources by appealing to the social worth of the candidates. Before appealing to the notion of social worth, however, the committee took several other factors into account. Upon the advice of physicians, persons over forty-five years old and very young children were automatically excluded from consideration. These persons, it was thought, would not respond as well to dialysis. Children, for example, may not mature physically on dialysis and may have a difficult time sticking to the diet. Also, children would require much more care for a longer period of time. The committee also excluded those who were not residents of Washington. This was done because the hospital received much of its funding from state taxes. Washingtonians were expecially entitled to the benefits of the hospital, it was thought.

Of the remaining candidates, the persons selected were those thought to have the greatest social worth. Exactly how social worth was determined remains unclear. It is known, however, what sort of information the committee requested. The committee wanted to know the following about each of the prospective patients: the age, sex, marital status, number of dependents, income, emotional stability (especially the patient's capacity to accept treatment), nature of occupation, educational background, past performances and future potential.[21] The committee was not told the names of the candidates; if the prospective patients did not remain anonymous, the committee might be open to the charge of personal favoritism or bias. The information that the committee asked for was conveyed by the patient's physician. Bits and pieces of the committee's deliberations have been reported. It was said that the committee looked favorably on those who played an active role in a church. This, some members thought, was an indication of moral strength. And the evidence suggests that the committee tended to give preference to persons with many dependents and to those who were poor.

The work of the Seattle committee has been widely criticized.[22] The following are the most common objections that have been raised. First, the case for each patient was made by his or her doctor. But some people write better and argue more persuasively than others. And so how well and convincingly a patient's physician could write greatly affected that patient's chances of being chosen by the committee. Moreover, some people may be inclined to exaggerate when making such a case (to enhance the chances of his or her patient), while others will be scrupulously honest. And it is clear that these factors should not play a role in determining whether the patient receives a scarce medical resource. A physician is not hired because he or she can write well, argue, or is inclined to exaggerate. Second, some critics expressed the concern that any such committee will inevitably involve the promotion of bourgeois values. What underlies this criticism is the belief that our knowledge of social worth is very limited and that most of the criteria of social worth that have been proposed are hopelessly inadequate. One author, for example, sardonically noted that a patient coming before the Seattle committee would do well to father a great number of children and to throw away all of his money. Others quipped that a nonconformist such as Henry David Thoreau would not fare well if he lived in Seattle and had bad kidneys.[23] History is fraught with examples where a person's contemporaries castigated him or her, and only later generations appreciated the person's true worth. Finally, it is argued that the use of the social worth criterion is, inappropriately, a case of people "playing God." What this means, apparently, is that each person possesses an equal right to life and an equal right to the medical care necessary to maintain life. The sorts of decisions made by the Seattle committee run counter to this in that they suggest that the person supposed to possess more social worth possesses a greater right to the medical care in short supply. Thus, the critic charges, introducing the notion of social worth in such a context is totally inappropriate.

Before dismissing completely the social worth theory, though, it is advisable to examine a more detailed version of it.

## DISTRIBUTING SCARCE MEDICAL RESOURCES: AN APPEAL TO SOCIAL WORTH

In spite of the objections to the work of the Seattle committee, some have thought that the notion of social worth or utility must play some role in deciding who will receive scarce medical resources. Certainly in some medical contexts the notion of utility is appealed to. For example, in allocating money to fund research projects, officials consider how many people might be helped if the research is successful. So perhaps such considerations may be invoked in distributing medical resources too.

Nicholas Rescher has recently defended an approach to this problem that takes into account some considerations of social worth.[24] Rescher suggests that the process of choosing those who will receive scarce medical resources be divided into two stages. Different criteria are needed for each of these stages. The first stage is designed to narrow the field of applicants to a workable number. To accomplish this, what Rescher calls *criteria of inclusion* must be formulated. Persons who do not satisfy the criteria of inclusion will not be considered; they will be excluded. Persons who do satisfy the criteria of inclusion will be considered at the second stage; they are the serious candidates. How criteria of inclusion work is simple enough. Consider the admissions policy of a university. If, as is true of the best universities, a school receives far more applications than it has positions available, it is not feasible to examine carefully the credentials of each applicant. So a university may have certain requirements which function as criteria of inclusion. It may, for example, routinely refuse admission to anyone who scores below a certain level on the entrance examination. Or it may reject any student whose high school grade point average falls below a certain fixed mark. Following such a procedure, one is then able to examine the records of each of the remaining students very carefully on a case by case basis. When the field of applicants has been narrowed down to a workable number, one then needs additional criteria to choose who among them will receive the scarce resource. Criteria to be employed at this second stage are called by Rescher *criteria of comparison*. To continue the previous analogy, at this second stage a university might study carefully the applicant's letters of recommendation, his or her extracurricular activities, and the like.

To narrow the field of applicants for a scarce medical resource, Rescher suggests three criteria of inclusion. The first of these is what he calls the *constituency factor*.[25] It is a fact of life that most medical resources are available only in the institutional setting of the hospital. And sometimes hospitals or medical institutes have what might be called normal clientele boundaries; that is, some hospitals are set up to serve only certain patients, or at least to serve them first. Examples include veterans' hospitals, hospitals supported by certain churches, and hospitals supported through funds from the state. When allocating scarce medical resources, Rescher contends, a medical institution is justified in giving preference to those persons who are a part of its natural constituency. This, of course, is exactly what the Swedish Hospital did when it chose Washingtonians ahead of all others. The rationale for this presumably is that those who are a part of the hospital's natural clientele have a special entitlement to the resources of that institution.

The second criterion of inclusion proposed by Rescher is the *progress-of-science factor*.[26] It is important for the medical practitioner to learn as much as he or she can about how a certain drug or form of treatment will affect future patients. And it may be that certain types of scarce medical resources have never been given to certain patients. Thus it is important to learn how it will affect those persons; learning this can benefit many patients of the future. For example, it may be useful for the medical worker to determine how effective a certain medical resource is on persons over the age of sixty or persons with a negative Rh factor. This consideration may be taken into account in reducing the field of initial applicants.

Suppose that the results of previous treatments show that a given scarce medical resource is highly effective only for a certain class of patients. Suppose, for example, that only women under the age of forty or persons with a certain blood type can be treated effectively with the resource in question. If this is the case, Rescher says, it is appropriate to consider only those patients for whom the treatment is likely to be successful. This is the third criterion of inclusion, what is called the *prospect-of-success factor*.[27] Each of these factors, it is worth noting, is utilitarian or pragmatic in nature. The latter two, especially, are proposed with an eye toward maximizing the number of lives that can be saved.

Let us turn now to the criteria of comparison suggested by Rescher. There are five in all, the first two of which are medical in nature and the last three of which appeal to the notion of social worth. The first criterion of comparison is called the *relative-likelihood-of-*

*success factor.*[28] This, of course, is similar to the third criterion of inclusion. The difference, though, is that this involves a case by case comparison. Two patients may fall in the same general category, yet the severity of the medical problem of one patient may be greater than that of the other patient. If this is the case (and everything else is equal), then for medical reasons it makes sense to give the scarce medical resource to the patient who has the greater probability of being saved by it.

The *life-expectancy factor* is the second criterion of comparison put forward by Rescher.[29] This factor invites us to consider the patient's age and other aspects (that is, other than those to be treated by the scarce medical resource) of his or her medical condition. The idea behind this criterion is that those who have a longer life expectancy should be given preference. Thus if one patient is twenty-five years old, and a second is sixty-five years old, and if each has the medical problem at roughly the same degree of severity, then in case of a conflict the younger of the two should be given preference. His or her life expectancy is greater. Similarly, if the medical problem of each of two patients is roughly the same but one of these patients has an additional problem, say cancer, then the person without this additional complication should be saved first because his or her life expectancy is greater. The general idea behind this criterion is that a scarce medical resource is very valuable and should be given to those who will benefit the most from it. And those who will benefit the most are patients who will live many additional years because they are treated with the resource in question.

Rescher calls the third criterion of comparison the *family role factor.*[30] People are important to others as well as to themselves. In particular, the relationship between a person and his or her spouse, children, and parents is very important. Often members of a person's immediate family are financially and/or emotionally dependent on that person. It is appropriate to take this into account when distributing exotic lifesaving therapy, Rescher claims. If other things are equal, a mother with children dependent on her should be saved before a middle-aged bachelor. This is a utilitarian consideration; it appeals to the well-being of those other than the patients who will be directly affected by the decision.

The next criterion is the *potential future-contributions factor.*[31] In taking this factor into account, society must examine the candidates and try to determine who will be likely to render valuable services in the future. In making such a judgment the patient's age, talent, the importance of his or her job, the training the person has, and the past record of performance must be considered. Such a procedure is appropriate, the argument goes, because society is "investing" one of its scarce and valuable resources. Since, in investing this resource, society must choose among its citizens, it is entitled to a likely return. Thus this criterion counsels us to choose a brilliant surgeon over a common laborer, and a research physicist over a childless homemaker. Of course, it will often be difficult to determine who among other candidates will be likely to contribute the most. Clearly such judgments are quite fallible. But, that the judgments are often difficult to make is not reason for not trying to make them at all, Rescher argues.

Finally, Rescher's fifth criterion of comparison is the *past services-rendered factor*.[32] This is said to be a necessary correlate of the factor of prospective service. A society, like individuals, can incur a debt of gratitude. If someone has worked long and hard for the good of society, that person should be rewarded. Thus it is appropriate for society to give preference to those who have rendered significant services in the past when allocating scarce medical resources. In deciding whether to give a scarce medical resource to a "life-long" criminal or a retired nurse, then, the latter should be given preference because of the past services the person has rendered.

This system, as presented so far, is not complete. Clearly the five criteria of comparison can, on occasion, conflict. A method for handling such conflicts is needed. A number of possibilities come to mind. A hierarchical arrangement of the five criteria might be suggested. Thus someone might propose that the relative-likelihood-of-success factor is the most important and should take precedence over the other four, that the life-expectancy factor is the second most important, and so forth. Rescher himself says that as long as all five of the factors are taken into account there are many appropriate ways to settle possible conflicts. The method that he himself prefers is to give equal weight to the medical factors (that is, the likelihood-of-success and life-expectancy) and the extramedical factors (that is, the three social considerations). Of course, if equal weight is given to each of these sets, then the possibility of a tie still exists. The patient with the greatest likelihood of success may be a convicted criminal, and the person who has rendered or probably will render the greatest services to society may have a much lower probability of success. When this point is reached, Rescher suggests that a random method of selection be employed. To use the random method of selection at that stage has several advantages, Rescher maintains. It will be perceived to be more fair, rejected patients will feel less bitter, and those who have to deal with these cases will be relieved of at least some difficult decisions.

This, then, is a brief sketch of a method of allocating scarce medical resources that allows the notion of social worth to play a key role in the decisions to be made. Whether this system avoids the difficulties that were raised concerning the work of the Seattle committee is worth pondering. It appears that the objection that such a system inappropriately promotes bourgeois values still has some force. Nonconformists are not likely to be treated well in such a system; yet it is just such people who are often judged to be great when the verdict of history has been rendered. Some have also suggested that this system violates the fundamental western belief in the equality and intrinisic worth of all human beings. The system wrongly suggests that a great surgeon is a better person than a common laborer, the critic charges. Whether there are plausible responses to these objections is a matter for the reader to consider. For now, let us turn to an alternative system, one which purports to avoid these difficulties.

## DISTRIBUTING SCARCE MEDICAL RESOURCES: THE LOTTERY METHOD

Many have rejected the view that scarce medical resources ought to be allocated on the basis of utilitarian considerations or those of social worth. The most popular alternative to this position is the lottery method. Defenders of this view advocate that scarce medical resources be distributed by using some random method. Whether a candidate receives the scarce medical resource in question should be a matter of luck. There are different ways that such a method might be instituted. One way would be to have an actual lottery. Another way would be to adopt the policy "first come, first served." Under the latter system whether a patient receives the scarce medical resource in question depends on when that patient happens to need it and how many others have already requested it, and these are matters of luck.

The lottery method has been defended by several as the most appropriate way of allocating scarce medical resources. Here one defense of this method, offered by James Childress, will be examined.[33] Childress, like Rescher, advocates a two-step procedure. That is, the selection of recipients of scarce lifesaving medical resources should proceed in two different stages. The first stage (corresponding to Rescher's criteria of inclusion) should reduce the field of applicants by appealing only to medical considerations. The judgments made at this first stage, then, are medical judgments and should be made by medical personnel. That the judgments are medical rather than moral does not mean that they will be easy, however. What determines whether a person is medically acceptable and is to be included among those to be considered at the second stage? Childress argues that if a person has a reasonable prospect of responding to the treatment then he or she should be regarded as medically acceptable. What counts as a reasonable prospect of responding to treatment is not easy to say, but what Childress seems to have in mind is a rough judgment of common sense that the person has a pretty good chance of benefiting if the treatment is administered. Childress also maintains that medical considerations should be used only at this first stage. Once the second state is reached, no finer distinctions on medical grounds should be appealed to. That is, once it has been determined that each of two persons has a good chance of benefiting from the treatment in question, one should not be chosen over the other because he or she has a better chance of being helped.[34]

Regarding the selection process at the second stage, Childress advocates that some version of the lottery method be used. The strategy that he follows is first to raise a number of difficulties with the view that appeals to social worth, and then to cite some positive considerations that support the method of random selection. Any method that attempts to distribute scarce medical resources by appealing to the social worth of the candidates is defective, Childress thinks. First, there is a problem in determining the relevant criteria of social value. At best, it will be difficult to formulate criteria of social value that are even remotely plausible. Second, our judgments about who is valuable to society change radically over the years. As has been noted, persons like Socrates and Thoreau were denigrated by their contemporaries, but are now regarded as great. Third, who is valuable to society depends in part on society's needs, and those needs are ever changing and difficult to predict. Oblivious to our wasteful use of energy, few persons in the 1960s would have ranked geologists and petroleum engineers as extremely valuable because of their contributions. Such judgments are apt to be different today. Finally, it is claimed that allocating scarce medical resources according to the social role a person plays violates our basic belief in the equality of people. Were we to employ such a method, we would be saying to a person that his or her social worth is contingent upon the contribution made to the collective good. This seems contrary to the ideals of western society.[35] These, then, are the major reasons for rejecting the appeal to social worth.

There are, though, positive reasons for accepting some method of random selection. First, Childress argues, unlike the method that appeals to social worth, a method of random selection expresses our belief in the equality of people and it preserves a significant degree of personal dignity. Since a method of random selection truly provides for equality of opportunity, the society that employs it is expressing to each of the candidates a belief in his or her equal worth. Second, Childress asserts that this method will do more than any of its competitors in promoting the relationship of trust between the physician and patient. In order for one person to trust another, Childress believes that there must be the expectation that he or she will deal fairly with all people. If a person is assured that in conflict situations involving the allocating of scarce medical resources a method of random selection will be used, that person can be sure of being treated fairly and impartially. Finally, Childress speculates that the attitude of those who are not selected to receive the scarce medical resource will be much better if the reason is the luck of the draw rather than that they are judged to lack social worth.[36]

Childress does recommend that in implementing the method of random selection (at the second stage) that society adopt the policy of "first come, first served." Such a policy would work in the following way. Persons who passed the test of the first stage would be those whom physicians judged would have a good chance of benefiting from the scarce medical resource. If the resource were available at that time, be it a dialysis machine, an organ for transplantation, or whatever, the patient would be permitted to use it. If the resource were not available, then the patient would be in line, as it were, awaiting his or her turn. Should the resource become available while the patient can still benefit from it, then he or she is given access to it. Thus whether those who are medically acceptable receive the scarce medical resource in question depends on luck.

Once the lottery method is understood there is a temptation to look for exceptions, cases where a deliberate decision should be made instead of allowing the matter to be settled by chance. Childress himself is willing to allow for one exception.[37] He suggests that it would be appropriate to give preferential treatment to someone who is practically indispensable for a society, for example, the President in a grave national emergency. The difficulty, of course, is that allowing for one exception may open Pandora's box; once the first is allowed, there will be no end to the matter and all of the merits of the lottery method will have been lost.

In any case, some have charged that there are surely a number of situations in which it is irrational to use a method of random selection. These are situations in which a deliberate choice is called for. Consider the following cases.[38] First, suppose an emergency situation exists. A disaster has struck in the area. There are many people in need of immediate help and very few to give it. In this case, one of the scarce medical resources is the time and energy of the medical workers. Who should be treated first in such a situation? Should some version of the lottery method be adopted? Clearly it should not, critics argue. In a situation like this it is much more rational to treat first those persons who can be restored quickly. This will provide medical workers with additional help even if the patients are laymen. And certainly if some of the people in need of help are physicians or nurses, they should be treated first. This is not because they are "better" than the others; rather they are needed in order to save as many patients as possible.

Second, consider a situation in which a number of persons are stranded at sea. There are too many for the lifeboat to support, so some must be thrown overboard or all will die. This is like a situation involving the allocation of scarce medical resources in that the decision to be made is a life-or-death decision. Should the lottery method be used here? Again, critics have argued that it should not be employed. In particular, it is claimed, it would be irrational to include in a lottery those who are skilled in matters of navigation. After all, without them the chances are good that no one will be saved. So again there is an exception to the rule (favored by those who defend the lottery method) that no one should receive special treatment in these life-or-death situations.

Third, consider an actual historical case.[39] In 1943 there was a short supply of penicillin for the U.S. Armed Forces in North Africa. There were two groups of soldiers who could have benefited from its use: those who had venereal disease and those who had infected battle wounds. A decision had to be made concerning the allocation of the penicillin. Some argued that the wounded should be given priority on moral grounds. Perhaps what they had in mind was that those with venereal disease were more directly responsible for their plight. The medical officer in charge, however, argued that those with venereal disease should be treated. His reasoning was that they could be restored to active duty more quickly, thus better enabling the group to achieve its purpose. Since this is desirable, critics contend, this is yet another situation where it would be inappropriate to use the lottery method.

Finally, suppose that among those who are medically acceptable (in Childress's sense) are persons of questionable moral worth, for example, the proverbial mass murderer. If Charles Manson or Richard

Speck were among those who needed a scarce medical resource—say, an organ for transplantation—and who would probably benefit from it, would society really want to give such a person an equal opportunity to receive it? Granted, making comparative judgments of moral worth is a difficult task. But the extreme cases envisioned here are cases where society surely does feel confident about such judgments.

If one is persuaded by some or all of these cases, then there are two alternatives. The lottery method can be rejected as unacceptable and some other method can be adopted instead, or exceptions can be made to the general policy that each medically suitable patient must be given equal opportunity to receive the scarce medical resource in question. The difficulty with the latter move is that there must be a *principled* basis for allowing such exceptions; this cannot be done on an *ad hoc* basis merely to accommodate conflicting intuitions. The problem is even worse because the principled basis for allowing for these exceptions cannot be an appeal to social worth; if that were the basis, advocates of the lottery method would have conceded their case to defenders of the social worth theory.

The two views discussed here—the social worth theory and the lottery method—are the most widely held policies for distributing scarce medical resources. Only one other position has received much notice: when not all can be saved, no one should be saved.[40] This view, however, has few advocates and, on its face, seems not very plausible. The moral problem of how best to allocate scarce medical resources is especially worrisome because we realize that it is unavoidable and because the criticisms of each of the two major positions have a ring of plausibility. This creates a difficulty. We know that we must deal with the problem, yet we are acutely aware of the inadequacies of the usual ways of doing so. This problem is like so many of the others that we encounter in medical ethics. Through careful analysis, we can come to understand the major positions and the principal weaknesses of them. The challenge is to formulate an acceptable view on the basis of this knowledge.

## SUMMARY

Some medical resources are in short supply. When this is the case, steps must be taken to procure more of that resource. Cadaver organs are one type of scarce medical resource. There are three different policies that might be adopted for obtaining cadaver organs: the giving policy, the trading policy, and the taking policy. Each of these policies has certain advantages and certain disadvantages. Of the three, the giving policy places the least burden on people and respects the autonomy of individuals; unfortunately it has not been successful in generating an adequate supply of organs. The taking policy will provide the greatest supply of cadaver organs, but it forces a person to benefit others and is a policy that can be easily abused.

Some medical resources are renewable and must be obtained from living human beings. Blood and bone marrow are two examples. Among the policies that might be adopted for obtaining these resources are the free market system, the donorship system, the taxation system, and the penalty system. Judging these policies by the criteria of cost, quality of the resource obtained, efficiency, and moral acceptability, many have claimed that the donorship system is preferable. Of course, such a claim is controversial, and whether that system can provide an adequate supply is also debatable.

How scarce medical resources ought to be distributed is another moral problem. Decisions concerning such matters are often life-and-death ones. Two theories on this issue were examined. According to each of these views the procedure for allocating scarce medical resources should be a two-step one. The first step is designed to narrow the field of applicants to a workable number. Each of the competing theories agrees that only medical factors should be appealed to at this stage. Only persons who are likely to benefit from receiving the scarce resource should be considered seriously. At the second stage, however, the two theories differ. Nicholas Rescher defends a theory which recommends that scarce medical resources be allocated on utilitarian grounds. Among the medically qualified candidates, preference should be given to those who are likely to live longer, who have dependents, who are likely to contribute more to society in the future, and who have contributed more in the past. James Childress rejects such considerations. Instead, he argues that one should employ a random method for deciding who, among the medically qualified, should receive the scarce medical resource.

## CASE STUDY

You are the head of a small hospital in an isolated region of Alaska serving a small mining town and a nearby Army chemical and biological warfare unit. There is an accident and a newly developed nerve gas is released. In your judgment, a number of people affected by the accident require immediate hospitalization in your Intensive Care Unit (ICU). This unit normally has two beds. You can squeeze in a third one, although it will take an Army electrician four hours to make the appropriate hookups and jury rig the proper instrumentation. No more beds can be added. There is one person already in the ICU—Bill Marconi, an 87-year-old white male attempting to recover from his fifth myocardial infarction (death of tissues in the cardiac muscle resulting from the formation of a clot in the coronary arterial system). He has also suffered a series of massive strokes which has left his right arm and both legs paralyzed. The following people require hospitalization in the ICU:

James Soon: He is an 18-year-old male Oriental in otherwise excellent health. You believe he is virtually certain to recover with treatment because of a differential effect of the nerve gas on Orientals. However, he was nearest to the tank when the gas was released and is not likely to survive otherwise. He is unemployed, has a history of juvenile delinquency, and is on trial for attempted rape while AWOL.

George Preston: He is a 59-year-old white male with a history of early anginal pains. He is the senior senator from California and is on an inspection tour. It is believed that he has an excellent chance of being elected President in the next election. He is concerned with improving health care delivery and also has a flair for foreign affairs. He has no chance of survival without immediate hospitalization in the ICU, and only a poor chance with it.

Margaret Adams: She is a 30-year-old white female, in good health, divorced with three children, aged two, three, and five. She was stricken by accident, while participating in a protest against chemical and biological warfare along with her eldest daughter. She has a good chance of survival with ICU hospitalization; without hospitalization, she has no chance of survival.

Janey Adams: She is a five-year-old white female, in good health, and the daughter of Margaret Adams. She was recently evaluated as a super genius (180+ IQ). She has a good chance of survival with hospitalization and some chance of survival without the ICU.

Henrietta Stone: She is a 56-year-old black female with systemic lupus. This is not likely to interfere with her recovery from the nerve gas if she is treated promptly. She will otherwise not survive. She is a Nobel Prize winner and in Alaska working on her next book. She is quite rich and has announced that when she dies all of her money will go to fund research on lupus.

On the basis of the information given, decide who should be placed in the ICU.[41]

## Discussion Questions

1.  Suppose that the committee from the Swedish Hospital in Seattle were assigned to this case. Which of the candidates would they admit to the ICU and why?
2.  If we employ the criteria for allocating scarce medical resources suggested by Rescher, which candidates would be favored and why?
3.  If we employ the criteria for allocating scarce medical resources defended by Childress, which candidates would be admitted to the ICU and why?
4.  If you were the physician in this case and had to make the decision, what would you do?

## SUGGESTIONS FOR FURTHER READING

James F. Childress, "Rationing of Medical Treatment," in Warren T. Reich (ed.), *Encyclopedia of Bioethics* (New York: The Free Press, 1978), pp. 1414-1419.

James F. Childress, "Who Shall Live When Not All Can Live?" *Soundings*, Vol. 43 (1970), pp. 339-355.

Andrew L. Jameton, "Organ Donation: Ethical Issues," in Warren T. Reich (ed.), *Encylcopedia of Bioethics* (New York: The Free Press, 1978), pp. 1169-1173.

James L. Muyskens, "An Alternative Policy for Obtaining Cadaver Organs for Transplantation," *Philosopy & Public Affairs*, Vol. 8 (1978), pp. 88-99.

Paul Ramsey, *The Patient as Person* (New Haven, Conn.: Yale University Press, 1970), pp. 198-215 and 239-266.

Nicholas Rescher, "The Allocation of Exotic Medical Lifesaving Therapy," in Samuel Gorovitz *et al.* (eds.), *Moral Problems in Medicine* (Englewood Cliffs: Prentice-Hall, 1976), pp. 522-535.

Robert M. Veatch, *Death, Dying, and the Biological Revolution* (New Haven, Conn.: Yale University Press, 1976), pp. 249-276.

## NOTES

1.  Robert M. Veatch, *Death, Dying, and the Biological Revolution* (New Haven, Conn.: Yale University Press, 1976), p. 251.

2. Veatch, *Death, Dying, and the Biological Revolution*, p. 251.
3. These possibilities are discussed by James L. Muyskens in "An Alternative Policy for Obtaining Cadaver Organs for Transplantation," *Philosophy & Public Affairs*, Vol. 9 (1978), pp. 88-99. Much of my presentation in this selection is borrowed from this excellent article.
4. See Veatch, *Death, Dying, and the Biological Revolution*, pp. 269-270 and pp. 273-276. See also, Muyskens, "An Alternative Policy for Obtaining Cadaver Organs for Transplantation," pp. 89-90.
5. See Muyskens, "An Alternative Policy for Obtaining Cadaver Organs for Transplantation," p. 90.
6. No matter which policy is being discussed, those whose organs are used are called donors. Strictly speaking, when talking about the trading and taking policies, the term "donor" is out of place. This traditional term shall continue to be used, though calling the persons "contributors" would be more accurate.
7. These first two objections are discussed in Paul Ramsey, *The Patient as Person* (New Haven, Conn.: Yale University Press, 1970), p. 210.
8. See Veatch, *Death, Dying, and the Biological Revolution*, pp. 268-269.
9. The defense that I sketch here is presented in Muyskens, "An Alternative Policy for Obtaining Cadaver Organs for Transplantation," pp. 94-98.
10. This argument is presented by Muyskens, "An Alternative Policy for Obtaining Cadaver Organs for Transplantation," pp. 97-98.
11. A case that raises this question is presented in Robert M. Veatch, *Case Studies in Medical Ethics* (Cambridge, Mass.: Harvard University Press, 1977), pp. 319-325.
12. Several articles, reprinted in Samuel Gorovitz *et al.* (eds.), *Moral Problems in Medicine* (Englewood Cliffs, New Jersey: Prentice-Hall, 1976), have greatly influenced my presentation of this topic. They are the following: Richard M. Titmuss, "Why Give to Strangers?" pp. 500-504; A.J. Culyer, "Letters: Ethics and Economics in Blood Supply," pp. 505-506; Peter Singer, "Altruism and Commerce," pp. 507-510; and Robert M. Solow, "Blood and Thunder," pp. 510-521.
13. See especially the articles mentioned in note 12 above.
14. See Soslow, "Blood and Thunder," pp. 513-514 and p. 517.
15. Here one is reminded of the two positions that might be taken regarding the use of people who volunteer to be experimental subjects only because of the abjectness of their social conditions. See the discussion of the Willowbrook case in Chapter Four, pp. 106-107.
16. See Singer, "Altruism and Commerce," p. 510.
17. See Bernard Gaver, "Blood Money: The Donor Industry," *Parade*, December 2, 1979, p. 5.
18. The process of plasmapheresis is used to separate the plasma and the red cells. The red cells may then be reinjected into the contributor. If a person's red cells are returned, that person can safely contribute more frequently.
19. One of the cases introduced in Chapter Two, pp. 24-26, involves the issue of allocating a scarce medical resource and is designed to show that such problems are unavoidable.
20. For a discussion of this case, see Paul Ramsey, *The Patient as Person*, pp. 242-248.
21. See Ramsey, *The Patient as Person*, p. 246.

22. See Shana Alexander, "They Decide Who Lives, Who Dies," *Life*, November 9, 1962, pp. 102-110 and pp. 115-128. See also, David Sanders and Jesse Dukeminier, Jr., "Medical Advance and Legal Lag: Hemodialysis and Kidney Transplantation," *U.C.L.A. Law Review*, Vol. 15 (February, 1968). Many of these criticisms are noted by Ramsey, *The Patient as Person*, pp. 246-249.

23. The former claim is made by Shana Alexander, "They Decide Who Lives, Who Dies"; the latter, by David Sanders and Jesse Dukeminier, "Medical Advance and Legal Lag."

24. Nicholas Rescher, "The Allocation of Exotic Medical Lifesaving Therapy," in *Moral Problems in Medicine*, pp. 522-535.

25. Rescher, "The Allocation of Exotic Medical Lifesaving Therapy," pp. 525-526.

26. Rescher, "The Allocation of Exotic Medical Lifesaving Therapy," p. 526.

27. Rescher, "The Allocation of Exotic Medical Lifesaving Therapy," p. 526.

28. Rescher, "The Allocation of Exotic Medical Lifesaving Therapy," p. 527.

29. Rescher, "The Allocation of Exotic Medical Lifesaving Therapy," p. 527.

30. Rescher, "The Allocation of Exotic Medical Lifesaving Therapy," p. 528.

31. Rescher, "The Allocation of Exotic Medical Lifesaving Therapy," p. 528.

32. Rescher, "The Allocation of Exotic Medical Lifesaving Therapy," p. 529.

33. James F. Childress, "Who Shall Live When Not All Can Live?" *Soundings*, Vol. 43 (1970), pp. 339-355. Paul Ramsey, in *The Patient as Person*, pp. 252-259, also defends the lottery method.

34. Childress, "Who Shall Live When Not All Can Live?" pp. 343-344.

35. Childress articulates these criticisms in "Who Shall Live When Not All Can Live?" pp. 344-347.

36. Childress spells out these advantages in "Who Shall Live When Not All Can Live?" pp. 348-352.

37. Childress, "Who Shall Live When Not All Can Live?" pp. 353-354.

38. Most of these points are discussed by Paul Ramsey, *The Patient as Person*, pp. 255-259.

39. This is discussed by Paul A. Freund, "Organ Transplants: Ethical and Legal Problems," in *Moral Problems in Medicine*, pp. 537-538.

40. This view is discussed but rejected by Ramsey, *The Patient as Person*, pp. 259-266. For a defense of this position, see Edmund Cahn, *The Moral Decision* (Bloomington, Indiana: Indiana University Press, 1955), pp. 61-71.

41. This case is presented in Marc D. Basson (ed.), *Ethics, Humanism, and Medicine* (New York: Alan R. Liss, Inc., 1980), pp. 151-152. This case is reprinted with the permission of Alan R. Liss, Inc. and the editor.

# Appendix

## Codes of Ethics

### THE HIPPOCRATIC OATH[1]

I swear by Apollo Physician and Asclepius and Hygieia and Panaceia and all the gods and goddesses, making them my witness, that I will fulfil according to my ability and judgment this oath and this covenant:

To hold him who has taught me this art as equal to my parents and to live my life in partnership with him, and if he is in need of money to give him a share of mine, and to regard his offspring as equal to my brothers in male lineage and to teach them this art—if they desire to learn it—without fee and covenant; to give a share of precepts and oral instruction and all other learning to my sons and to the sons of him who has instructed me and to pupils who have signed the covenant and have taken an oath according to the medical law, but to no one else.

I will apply dietetic measures for the benefit of the sick according to my ability and judgment; I will keep them from harm and injustice.

I will neither give a deadly drug to anybody if asked for it, nor will I make a suggestion to this effect. Similarly I will not give to a woman an abortive remedy. In purity and holiness I will guard my life and my art.

I will not use the knife, not even on sufferers from stone, but will withdraw in favor of such men as are engaged in this work.

Whatever houses I may visit, I will come for the benefit of the sick, remaining free of all intentional injustice, of all mischief and in particular of sexual relations with both female and male persons, be they free or slaves.

What I may see or hear in the course of the treatment or even outside of the treatment in regard to the life of men, which on no account one must spread abroad, I will keep to myself holding such things shameful to be spoken about.

If I fulfil this oath and do not violate it, may it be granted to me to enjoy life and art, being honored with fame among all men for all time to come; if I transgress it and swear falsely, may the opposite of all this be my lot.

## AMERICAN MEDICAL ASSOCIATION
## PRINCIPLES OF MEDICAL ETHICS[2]

*Preamble.* These principles are intended to aid physicians individually and collectively in maintaining a high level of ethical conduct. They are not laws but standards by which a physician may determine the propriety of his conduct in his relationship with patients, with colleagues, with members of allied professions, and with the public.

*Section 1.* The principal objective of the medical profession is to render service to humanity with full respect for the dignity of man. Physicians should merit the confidence of patients entrusted to their care, rendering to each a full measure of service and devotion.

*Section 2.* Physicians should strive continually to improve medical knowledge and skill, and should make available to their patients and colleagues the benefits of their professional attainments.

*Section 3.* A physician should practice a method of healing founded on a scientific basis; and he should not voluntarily associate professionally with anyone who violates this principle.

*Section 4.* The medical profession should safeguard the public and itself against physicians deficient in moral character or professional competence. Physicians should observe all laws, uphold the dignity and honor of the profession and accept its self-imposed disciplines. They should expose, without hesitation, illegal or unethical conduct of fellow members of the profession.

*Section 5.* A physician may choose whom he will serve. In an emergency, however, he should render service to the best of his ability. Having undertaken the care of a patient, he may not neglect him; and unless he has been discharged he may discontinue his services only after giving adequate notice. He should not solicit patients.

*Section 6.* A physician should not dispose of his services under terms or conditions which tend to interfere with or impair the free and complete exercise of his medical judgment and skill or tend to cause a deterioration of the quality of medical care.

*Section 7.* In the practice of medicine a physician should limit the source of his professional income to medical services actually rendered by him, or under his supervision, to his patients. His fee should be commensurate with the services rendered and the patient's ability to pay. He should neither pay nor receive a commission for referral of patients. Drugs, remedies or appliances may be dispensed or supplied by the physician provided it is in the best interests of the patient.

*Section 8.* A physician should seek consultation upon request; in doubtful or difficult cases; or whenever it appears that the quality of medical service may be enhanced thereby.

*Section 9.* A physician may not reveal the confidences entrusted to him in the course of medical attendance, or the deficiencies he may observe in the character of patients, unless he is required to do so by law or unless it becomes necessary in order to protect the welfare of the individual or of the community.

*Section 10.* The honored ideals of the medical profession imply that the responsibilities of the physician extend not only to the individual, but also to society where these responsibilities deserve his interest and participation in activities which have the purpose of improving both the health and well-being of the individual and the community.

## DECLARATION OF GENEVA[3]

Medical vow adopted by the General Assembly of The World Medical Association at Geneva, Switzerland, September 1948, and amended by the 22nd World Medical Assembly, Sydney, Australia, August 1968.

At the Time of Being Admitted as a Member of the Medical Profession:

I solemnly pledge myself to consecrate my life to the service of humanity.

I will give to my teachers the respect and gratitude which is their due;

I will practice my profession with conscience and dignity;

The health of my patient will be my first consideration;

I will respect the secrets which are confided in me; even after the patient has died.

I will maintain by all the means in my power, the honor and the noble traditions of the medical profession;

My colleagues will be my brothers;

I will not permit considerations of religion, nationality, race, party politics or social standing to intervene between my duty and my patient;

I will maintain the utmost respect for human life, from the time of conception; even under threat, I will not use my medical knowledge contrary to the laws of humanity.

## INTERNATIONAL CODE OF NURSING ETHICS[4]

Professional nurses minister to the sick, assume responsibility for creating a physical, social and spiritual environment which will be conducive to recovery, and stress the prevention of illness and promotion of health by teaching and example. They render health-service to the individual, the family, and the community and coordinate their services with members of other health professions.

Service to mankind is the primary function of nurses and the reason for the existence of the nursing profession. Need for nursing service is universal. Professional nursing service is therefore unrestricted by considerations of nationality, race, creed, colour, politics, or social status.

Inherent in the code is the fundamental concept that the nurse believes in the essential freedoms of mankind and in the preservation of human life.

The profession recognizes that an international code cannot cover in detail all the activities and relationships of nurses, some of which are conditioned by personal philosophies and beliefs.

1.  The fundamental responsibility of the nurse is threefold: to conserve life, to alleviate suffering, and to promote health.
2.  The nurse must maintain at all times the highest standards of nursing care and of professional conduct.
3.  The nurse must not only be well prepared to practise but must maintain her knowledge and skill at a consistently high level.
4.  The religious beliefs of a patient must be respected.
5.  Nurses hold in confidence all personal information entrusted to them.
6.  A nurse recognizes not only the responsibilities but the limitations of her or his professional functions; recommends or gives medical treatment without medical orders only in emergencies and reports such action to a physician at the earliest possible moment.
7.  The nurse is under an obligation to carry out the physician's orders intelligently and loyally and to refuse to participate in unethical procedures.
8.  The nurse sustains confidence in the physician and other members of the health team: incompetence or unethical conduct of associates should be exposed but only to the proper authority.
9.  A nurse is entitled to just remuneration and accepts only such compensation as the contract, actual or implied, provides.
10. Nurses do not permit their names to be used in connection with the advertisement of products or with any other form of self advertisement.

11. The nurse cooperates with and maintains harmonious relationships with members of other professions and with her or his nursing colleagues.
12. The nurse in private life adheres to standards of personal ethics which reflect credit upon her profession.
13. In personal conduct nurses should not knowingly disregard the accepted patterns of behaviour of the community in which they live and work.
14. A nurse should participate and share responsibility with other citizens and other health professions in promoting efforts to meet the health needs of the public—local, state, national and international.

## PATIENT'S BILL OF RIGHTS[5]

The American Hospital Association presents a Patient's Bill of Rights with the expectation that observance of these rights will contribute to more effective patient care and greater satisfaction for the patient, his physician, and the hospital organization. Further, the Association presents these rights in the expectation that they will be supported by the hospital on behalf of its patients, as an integral part of the healing process. It is recognized that a personal relationship between the physician and the patient is essential for the provision of proper medical care. The traditional physician–patient relationship takes on a new dimension when care is rendered within an organizational structure. Legal precedent has established that the institution itself also has a responsibility to the patient. It is in recognition of these factors that these rights are affirmed.

1. The patient has the right to considerate and respectful care.
2. The patient has the right to obtain from his physician complete current information concerning his diagnosis, treatment, and prognosis in terms the patient can be reasonably expected to understand. When it is not medically advisable to give such information to the patient, the information should be made available to an appropriate person in his behalf. He has the right to know by name, the physician responsible for coordinating his care.
3. The patient has the right to receive from his physician information necessary to give informed consent prior to the start of any procedure and/or treatment. Except in emergencies, such information for informed consent, should include but not necessarily be limited to the specific procedure and/or treatment, the medically

significant risks involved, and the probable duration of incapacitation. Where medically significant alternatives for care or treatment exist, or when the patient requests information concerning medical alternatives, the patient has the right to such information. The patient also has the right to know the name of the person responsible for the procedures and/or treatment.

4. The patient has the right to refuse treatment to the extent permitted by law, and to be informed of the medical consequences of his action.

5. The patient has the right to every consideration of his privacy concerning his own medical care program. Case discussion, consultation, examination, and treatment are confidential and should be conducted discreetly. Those not directly involved in his care must have the permission of the patient to be present.

6. The patient has the right to expect that all communications and records pertaining to his care should be treated as confidential.

7. The patient has the right to expect that within its capacity a hospital must make reasonable response to the request of a patient for services. The hospital must provide evaluation, service and/or referral as indicated by the urgency of the case. When medically permissible a patient may be transferred to another facility only after he has received complete information and explanation concerning the needs for and alternatives to such a transfer. The institution to which the patient is to be transferred must first have accepted the patient for transfer.

8. The patient has the right to obtain information as to any relationship of his hospital to other health care and educational institutions insofar as his care is concerned. The patient has the right to obtain information as to the existence of any professional relationships among individuals, by name, who are treating him.

9. The patient has the right to be advised if the hospital proposes to engage in or perform human experimentation affecting his care or treatment. The patient has the right to refuse to participate in such research projects.

10. The patient has the right to expect reasonable continuity of care. He has the right to know in advance what appointment times and physicians are available and where. The patient has the right to expect that the hospital will provide a mechanism whereby he is informed by his physician or a delegate of the physician of the patient's continuing health care requirements following discharge.

11. The patient has the right to examine and receive an explanation of his bill regardless of source of payment.

12. The patient has the right to know what hospital rules and regulations apply to his conduct as a patient.

No catalogue of rights can guarantee for the patient the kind of treatment he has a right to expect. A hospital has many functions to perform, including the prevention and treatment of disease, the education of both health professionals and patients, and the conduct of clinical research. All these activities must be conducted with an overriding concern for the patient, and, above all, the recognition of his dignity as a human being. Success in achieving this recognition assures success in the defense of the rights of the patient.

## THE NUREMBERG CODE[6]

1. The voluntary consent of the human subject is *absolutely* essential.
   This means that the person involved should have legal capacity to give consent; should be so situated as to be able to exercise free power of choice, without the intervention of any element of force, fraud, deceit, duress, overreaching, or other ulterior form of constraint or coercion; and should have sufficient knowledge and comprehension of the elements of the subject matter involved as to enable him to make an understanding and enlightened decision. This latter element requires that before the acceptance of an affirmative decision by the experimental subject there should be made known to him the nature, duration, and purpose of the experiment; the method and means by which it is to be conducted; all inconveniences and hazards reasonably to be expected; and the effects upon his health or person which may possibly come from his participation in the experiment.
   The duty and responsibility for ascertaining the quality of the consent rests upon each individual who initiates, directs, or engages in the experiment. It is a personal duty and responsibility which may not be delegated to another with impunity.
2. The experiment should be such as to yield fruitful results for the good of society, unprocurable by other methods or means of study, and not random and unnecessary in nature.
3. The experiment should be so designed and based on the results of animal experimentation and a knowledge of the natural history of the disease or other problem under study that the anticipated results will justify the performance of the experiment.
4. The experiment should be so conducted as to avoid all unnecessary physical and mental suffering and injury.

5. No experiment should be conducted where there is an *a priori* reason to believe that death or disabling injury will occur; except, perhaps, in those experiments where the experimental physicians also serve as subjects.

6. The degree of risk to be taken should never exceed that determined by the humanitarian importance of the problem to be solved by the experiment.

7. Proper preparations should be made and adequate facilities provided to protect the experimental subject against even remote possibilities of injury, disability, or death.

8. The experiment should be conducted only by scientifically qualified persons. The highest degree of skill and care should be required through all stages of the experiment of those who conduct or engage in the experiment.

9. During the course of the experiment the human subject should be at liberty to bring the experiment to an end if he has reached the physical or mental state where continuation of the experiment seems to him to be impossible.

10. During the course of the experiment the scientist in charge must be prepared to terminate the experiment at any stage, if he has probable cause to believe, in the exercise of the good faith, superior skill, and careful judgment required of him that a continuation of the experiment is likely to result in injury, disability, or death to the experimental subject.

## DECLARATION OF HELSKINKI[7]

Recommendations guiding medical doctors in biomedical research involving human subjects, adopted by the 18th World Medical Assembly, Helsinki, Finland, 1964, and revised by the 19th World Medical Assembly, Tokyo, Japan, 1975.

### Introduction

It is the mission of the medical doctor to safeguard the health of the people. His or her knowledge and conscience are dedicated to the fulfillment of this mission.

The Declaration of Geneva of the World Medical Association binds the doctor with the words, "The health of my patient will be my first consideration," and the International Code of Medical Ethics declares that, "Any act or advice which could weaken physical or mental resistance of a human being may be used only in his interest."

The purpose of biomedical research involving human subjects must be to improve diagnostic, therapeutic and prophylactic procedures and the understanding of the aetiology and pathogenesis of disease.

In current medical practice most diagnostic, therapeutic or prophylactic procedures involve hazards. This applies *a fortiori* to biomedical research.

Medical progress is based on research which ultimately must rest in part on experimentation involving human subjects.

In the field of biomedical research a fundamental distinction must be recognized between medical research in which the aim is essentially diagnostic or therapeutic for a patient, and medical research, the essential object of which is purely scientific and without direct diagnostic or therapeutic value to the person subjected to the research.

Special caution must be exercised in the conduct of research which may affect the environment, and the welfare of animals used for research must be respected.

Because it is essential that the results of laboratory experiments be applied to human beings to further scientific knowledge and to help suffering humanity, The World Medical Association has prepared the following recommendations as a guide to every doctor in biomedical research involving human subjects. They should be kept under review in the future. It must be stressed that the standards as drafted are only a guide to physicians all over the world. Doctors are not relieved from criminal, civil and ethical responsibilities under the laws of their own countries.

## I.  Basic Principles

1.  Biomedical research involving human subjects must conform to generally accepted scientific principles and should be based on adequately performed laboratory and animal experimentation and on a thorough knowledge of the scientific literature.

2.  The design and performance of each experimental procedure involving human subjects should be clearly formulated in an experimental protocol which should be transmitted to a specially appointed independent committee for consideration, comment and guidance.

3.  Biomedical research involving human subjects should be conducted only by scientifically qualified persons and under the supervision of a clinically competent medical person. The respon-

sibility for the human subject must always rest with a medically qualified person and never rest on the subject of the research, even though the subject has given his or her consent.

4. Biomedical research involving human subjects cannot legitimately be carried out unless the importance of the objective is in proportion to the inherent risk to the subject.

5. Every biomedical research project involving human subjects should be preceded by careful assessment of predictable risks in comparison with forseeable benefits to the subject or to others. Concern for the interests of the subject must always prevail over the inest of science and society.

6. The right of the research subject to safeguard his or her integrity must always be respected. Every precaution should be taken to respect the privacy of the subject and to minimize the impact of the study on the subject's physical and mental integrity and on the personality of the subject.

7. Doctors should abstain from engaging in research projects involving human subjects unless they are satisfied that the hazards involved are believed to be predictable. Doctors should cease any investigation if the hazards are found to outweigh the potential benefits.

8. In publication of the results of his or her research, the doctor is obliged to preserve the accuracy of the results. Reports of experimentation not in accordance with the principles laid down in this Declaration should not be accepted for publication.

9. In any research on human beings, each potential subject must be adequately informed of the aims, methods, anticipated benefits and potential hazards of the study and the discomfort it may entail. He or she should be informed that he or she is at liberty to abstain from participation in the study and that he or she is free to withdraw his or her consent to participation at any time. The doctor should then obtain the subject's freely-given informed consent, preferably in writing.

10. When obtaining informed consent for the research project the doctor should be particularly cautious if the subject is in a dependent relationship to him or her or may consent under duress. In that case the informed consent should be obtained by a doctor who is now engaged in the investigation and who is completely independent of this official relationship.

11. In case of legal incompetence, informed consent should be obtained from the legal guardian in accordance with national legisla-

tion. Where physical or mental incapacity makes it impossible to obtain informed consent, or when the subject is a minor, permission from the responsible relative replaces that of the subject in accordance with national legislation.

12. The research protocol should always contain a statement of the ethical considerations involved and should indicate that the principles enunciated in the present Declaration are complied with.

## II. Medical Research Combined with Professional Care (Clinical Research)

1. In the treatment of the sick person, the doctor must be free to use a new diagnostic and therapeutic measure, if in his or her judgment it offers hope of saving life, reestablishing health or alleviating suffering.
2. The potential benefits, hazards and discomfort of a new method should be weighed against the advantages of the best current diagnostic and therapeutic methods.
3. In any medical study, every patient—including those of a control group, if any—should be assured of the best proven diagnostic and therapeutic method.
4. The refusal of the patient to participate in a study must never interfere with the doctor–patient relationship.
5. If the doctor considers it essential not to obtain informed consent, the specific reasons for this proposal should be stated in the experimental protocol for transmission to the independent committee (1, 2).
6. The doctor can combine medical research with professional care, the objective being the acquisition of new medical knowledge, only to the extent that medical research is justified by its potential diagnostic or therapeutic value for the patient.

## III. Non-therapeutic Biomedical Research Involving Human Subjects (Non-Clinical Biomedical Research)

1. In the purely scientific application of medical research carried out on a human being, it is the duty of the doctor to remain the protector of the life and health of that person on whom biomedical research is being carried out.
2. The subjects should be volunteers—either healthy persons or patients for whom the experimental design is not related to the patient's illness.

3. The investigator or the investigating team should discontinue the research if in his/her or their judgment it may, if continued, be harmful to the individual.

4. In research on man, the interest of science and society should never take precedence over considerations related to the wellbeing of the subject.

## AMERICAN MEDICAL ASSOCIATION ETHICAL GUIDELINES FOR CLINICAL INVESTIGATION[8]

The following guidelines are intended to aid physicians in fulfilling their ethical responsibilities when they engage in the clinical investigation of new drugs and procedures.

1. A physician may participate in clinical investigation only to the extent that his activities are a part of a systematic program competently designed, under accepted standards of scientific research, to produce data which is scientifically valid and significant.

2. In conducting clinical investigation, the investigator should demonstrate the same concern and caution for the welfare, safety and comfort of the person involved as is required of a physician who is furnishing medical care to a patient independent of any clinical investigation.

3. In clinical investigation *primarily for treatment—*
   A. The physician must recognize that the physician–patient relationship exists and that he is expected to exercise his professional judgment and skill in the best interest of the patient.
   B. Voluntary consent must be obtained from the patient, or from his legally authorized representative if the patient lacks the capacity to consent, following: (a) disclosure that the physician intends to use an investigational drug or experimental procedure, (b) a reasonable explanation of the nature of the drug or procedure to be used, risks to be expected, and possible therapeutic benefits, (c) an offer to answer any inquiries concerning the drug or procedure, and (d) a disclosure of alternative drugs or procedures that may be available.
      i. In exceptional circumstances and to the extent that disclosure of information concerning the nature of the drug or experimental procedure or risks would be expected to materially affect the health of the patient and would be

detrimental to his best interests, such information may be withheld from the patient. In such circumstances such information shall be disclosed to a responsible relative or friend of the patient where possible.

    ii.   Ordinarily, consent should be in writing, except where the physician deems it necessary to rely upon consent in other than written form because of the physical or emotional state of the patient.

    iii.  Where emergency treatment is necessary and the patient is incapable of giving consent and no one is available who has authority to act on his behalf, consent is assumed.

4.  In clinical investigation *primarily for the accumulation of scientific knowledge—*

    A.  Adequate safeguards must be provided for the welfare, safety and comfort of the subject.

    B.  Consent, in writing, should be obtained from the subject, or from his legally authorized representative if the subject lacks the capacity to consent, following: (a) a disclosure of the fact that an investigational drug or procedure is to be used, (b) a reasonable explanation of the nature of the procedure to be used and risks to be expected, and (c) an offer to answer any inquiries concerning the drug or procedure.

    C.  Minor or mentally incompetent persons may be used as subjects only if:

        i.   The nature of the investigation is such that mentally competent adults would not be suitable subjects.

        ii.  Consent, in writing, is given by a legally authorized representative of the subject under circumstances in which an informed and prudent adult would reasonably be expected to volunteer himself or his child as a subject.

    D.  No person may be used as a subject against his will.

# NOTES

1.  Reprinted with permission of the publisher from Owsei Temkin and C. Lilian Temkin (eds.), *Ancient Medicine: Selected Papers of Ludwig Edelstein* (Baltimore: Johns Hopkins University Press, 1967), p. 6.
2.  Reprinted with the permission of the American Medical Association.
3.  Reprinted with the permission of the World Medical Association.

4. Reprinted with permission from M.B. Etziony (ed.), *The Physician's Creed* (Springfield, Illinois: Charles C. Thomas, 1973). Copyright by the *Israel Journal of Medical Science*.
5. Reprinted with the permission of the American Hospital Association.
6. Reprinted from *Trials of War Criminals before the Nuremberg Military Tribunals*, (Washington, D.C.: U.S. Government Printing Office, 1948).
7. Reprinted with permission from the World Medical Association.
8. Reprinted with permission from the American Medical Association.

# Index